# Blacks and Aids

## Causes and Origins

**Samuel V. Duh**

**Sage Series on Race and Ethnic Relations**

v o l u m e    3

*For information address*:

SAGE Publications, Inc.
2455 Teller Road
Newbury Park, California 91320

SAGE Publications Ltd.
6 Bonhill Street
London EC2A 4PU
United Kingdom

SAGE Publications India Pvt. Ltd.
M-32 Market
Greater Kailash I
New Delhi 110 048 India

Printed in the United States of America

**Library of Congress Cataloging-in-Publication Data**

Duh, Samuel V.
    Blacks and AIDS: causes and origins / Samuel V. Duh.
        p.      cm.—(Sage series on race and ethnic relations; v. 3)
    Includes bibliographical references.
    ISBN 0-8039-4346-6 (cloth). —ISBN 0-8039-4347-4 (pbk.)
    1. AIDS (Disease)—Epidemiology.  2. AIDS (Diseases)—United
States.  3. Afro-Americans—Diseases.  4. Blacks—Diseases.
I. Title.  II. Series.
    [DNLM: 1. Acquired Immunodeficiency Syndrome—genetics.
2. Blacks.   WD 308 D869b]
RA 644.A25D84   1991
614.5′993—dc20
DNLM/DLC
for Library of Congress                                                91-15553
                                                                              CIP

**FIRST PRINTING, 1991**

Sage Production Editor: Michelle R. Starika

# Contents

# Foreword

AIDS is a tragic disease. It has perplexed the greatest minds in the global medical community. The search for the causes of AIDS and for cures has not only revealed much about how contemporary medical research is done but also has brought to light folk values, beliefs, and attitudes that can serve as windows into dominant American and other western cultures. One folk belief that has surfaced in the United States and abroad is that African-descent populations are primary carriers of epidemic (usually sexually transmitted) diseases. In past times and places, epidemic diseases such as venereal disease, yellow fever, and malaria were thought by many Europeans and Americans to have originated in the genes and/or cultures of African-descent populations. The same has been said, or at least thought about, the possible origins of AIDS.

In this fascinating and well-written book, Dr. Samuel Duh, a physician with extensive clinical and research experience on AIDS, introduces the race-linked explanation about the origins and spread of AIDS and explains why it is a serious misconception. As well, he offers thought-provoking environmental and physiological explanations about how and why AIDS spreads. His discussions shed interesting light on why nonaffluent African-Americans and Africans in certain continental subregions are AIDS victims in disproportionate numbers.

Duh's informed observations and his policy recommendations are bound to be important and stimulating food for thought about one of this century's most dismal public health problems—a problem that has become convoluted, unfortunately, by becoming entangled in that most dangerous myth: race.

John H. Stanfield II
*Series Editor*

# Preface

One of the success stories of organized medicine is the conquest, by the turn of the century, of many of the infectious diseases that had killed millions of people. The development of various vaccines and antibiotics made this possible. More important, advancement in environmental and economic conditions also affected this trend. In developed countries, at least, both the lay public and the medical community seemed to view such killer diseases as polio, measles, and influenza as things of the past. Then, suddenly, in the early 1980s, the world was beset with a killer infectious disease called *acquired immunodeficiency syndrome* (AIDS).

Initially, AIDS occurred mostly among male homosexuals. Subsequently, it was found in intravenous drug users, blood and blood product recipients, and, finally, heterosexuals. Current knowledge indicates that anybody can contract AIDS; it is found in almost every country and in almost every demographic group. However, the incidence and prevalence of AIDS are rather unevenly distributed. Black people are disproportionately affected: They have the highest rates of infection; they progress more quickly from HIV infection to acquisition of AIDS; and they die more quickly from the disease. Recent data indicate that the incidence is increasing more rapidly in blacks than in other racial/ethnic groups. Why are there such high rates and quick deaths among black people?

Much has been written about AIDS since its discovery in 1981. But there currently is no book available that comprehensively addresses the issue of AIDS in black populations. Such a book is urgently needed in light of the alarming incidence rates, and I decided to contribute to meeting that need.

The main issue addressed in this book is whether the disproportionately high rates of AIDS in blacks has a genetic basis. The issue is discussed in a comprehensive manner in terms of epidemiological, basic science, and clinical research data. The major topics discussed are the overall health status of blacks, the history and epidemiology of AIDS, transmission and pathogenesis, AIDS in Africa, genetic versus environmental basis of AIDS, and control measures.

But this is more than an "AIDS book." It deals with the psychosocial, socioeconomic, and cultural bases of the health status of blacks, which relate to adverse race/ethnic relationships involving long-standing discrimination and prejudice. The hypothesis is a seemingly simple one: The prevalence of AIDS is higher in blacks for the same reasons that the prevalence of heart disease, stroke, diabetes, hypertension, cancer, tuberculosis, syphilis, and so on is higher in blacks. Black people tend to have a lower socioeconomic status, which leads to lower health status, which in turn makes them susceptible to all kinds of diseases.

For decades, the health status of blacks has been lowered by physical and fiscal barriers. This trend is continued with the AIDS epidemic. Blacks are less involved in testing and counseling, research, and experimental drug protocol programs. Black AIDS patients tend to seek medical care later in the disease process. There are very few community-based organizations addressing AIDS in blacks; and, when they exist, they are less likely to secure funding from private sources.

The problem of AIDS has shed further light on the whole health care system, which puts certain population groups at a disadvantage. The approach to the control of AIDS in blacks, therefore, should be comprehensive, addressing all major issues affecting their health status. This is the aim and approach of this book. I will, therefore, discuss such seemingly unrelated subjects as epidemiology, microbiology, politics, and sociology. Regarding AIDS specifically, I will try to discuss all major topics— that is, epidemiology, transmission and pathogenesis, clinical presentation, and pharmacological treatment—which will serve as background for discussion of control measures.

Although a lot of technical information is presented, the language is simple enough that even basic microbiology should be comprehensible to the average reader. The book should be useful to physicians and other health care professionals, politicians, organizations and societies dealing with all aspects of AIDS, and individuals/organizations involved with race/ethnic relations. I hope this book will make a contribution to the control of AIDS worldwide.

# 1

# Introduction

From June 1981 to September 1990, 152,126 cases of acquired immunodeficiency syndrome (AIDS) were reported to the U.S. Centers for Disease Control (CDC, 1990). Reports of AIDS cases to the CDC have come from all 50 states and the District of Columbia. Most of the reported cases (55%) have occurred among white people. However, U.S. blacks are disproportionately represented in the cases relative to their representation in the U.S. population. Although blacks constitute 12% of the U.S. population, they account for 28% of AIDS cases. Furthermore, blacks account for 73% of the total AIDS cases in heterosexual men, 52% in women, and 55% in children.

More significant is the fact that the rate of AIDS cases is increasing among blacks. In February 1989, blacks constituted 26% of AIDS cases; as of September 1990, they constituted 28%. In addition, both documented studies and estimates have indicated the highest rate of HIV infection in blacks, making future cases of AIDS in that population even higher. Also, once exposed to the AIDS virus, blacks progress more quickly to full-blown AIDS, and the time from AIDS diagnosis to death is shorter for black patients. Finally, the number of AIDS cases and the HIV-infection rate in certain black African countries is quite alarming. And there is a general belief that AIDS (or the virus that causes AIDS) originated in Africa. Why the disproportionately high rates of AIDS in black populations? Why does HIV infection seem to be spreading so fast among black people? Why do blacks die so quickly from AIDS?

In the past several years, I have made many speeches to various groups, both health professionals and the lay public, on AIDS. One of the questions I am most often asked during these presentations

and on informal basis is where AIDS came from—seemingly for con-
firmation that AIDS originated in Africa. Another frequent question
is why blacks are disproportionately represented in the number of
AIDS cases. I have always responded by saying that nobody knows
*exactly* where or when the AIDS virus originated or *exactly* why there
is such a high rate of AIDS cases in black populations. I then offer
some epidemiological and clinical information to explain the trends.

There is no dispute over the fact that scientists have not yet found
all the answers regarding the AIDS epidemic. But a lot has been
learned about AIDS and the virus that causes it so that intelligent
guesses and speculations can be made about certain issues. One conclusion many people are drawing from such speculations is that the
AIDS virus originated in Africa. With AIDS supposedly killing millions of African blacks, and U.S. blacks having very high rates of
AIDS cases, some people are speculating that genetics may play a
role in the disease process.

In July 1987, I heard an interesting but rather disturbing comment
on the public television show *Tony Brown's Journal*. The show was
on AIDS in blacks, and a young black man asked the guest experts,
who were all black: Since AIDS is killing millions of African blacks,
and AIDS cases are disproportionately high among U.S. blacks, is it
not likely that the AIDS virus is being used as a biological warfare
for genocide against black populations? Tony Brown, the host of the
show, appeared as astounded by the question as I was and asked who
would be waging such warfare. The questioner's response: "The pow-
ers that be."

There is speculation that there may be something in the genetic
makeup of blacks that makes them more susceptible to the AIDS
virus. And at least the questioner above has suggested that the virus is
being selectively directed toward blacks. This confusion about
AIDS in black populations really reflects confusion about the
whole AIDS epidemic. Indeed, the speculation about who gets or
should get AIDS has undergone somewhat of an evolution.

When AIDS became a recognized health condition in 1981, it was
identified in male homosexuals. The first few cases were mostly in
white male homosexuals. Many people, including many from the
black community, viewed AIDS as a white homosexual disease. Then
cases were found in individuals who use illicit intravenous drugs. So
AIDS became the disease of people who indulge in unconventional
(some say "abnormal") behavior. Finally, it became clear that

minorities were disproportionately represented in the number of AIDS cases. The effect of this evolution is that mainstream society has tended to view AIDS as someone else's disease, and, because it does not affect them, they couldn't care less. Current scientific evidence has demonstrated that anybody can acquire and die from AIDS. Yet a large portion of society still views AIDS as someone else's disease. The end result is that people with AIDS have suffered from lack of sympathy, lack of support, and, in many cases, discrimination

Black people have historically suffered from all kinds of discrimination. If AIDS becomes a black people's disease, there is a real danger of it becoming one more basis for discrimination. But is there a reason even to consider the possibility that AIDS could be viewed by some as a black people's disease? In addition to epidemiological data showing higher rates of reported AIDS cases in blacks, all kinds of reports suggest this possibility.

Many articles in scientific journals have implied the possibility of a genetic basis of AIDS as it affects black people. A 1987 article in the British medical journal *Lancet* (Eales et al., 1987) stated that a particular gene that may predispose some to be AIDS carriers is higher in black Americans. Two different studies reported in *The New England Journal of Medicine* in 1987 (Diager & Brewton, 1987; Gilles et al., 1987) failed to confirm this finding, yet the earlier finding has been used in subsequent publications. A booklet on AIDS, published by the Harris County (Houston, Texas) Medical Society (1987) and distributed free to the public, states that the Gc1F gene occurs more frequently in blacks and may explain the higher AIDS rate in blacks.

Several individuals prominent in the AIDS "scene" have expressed concern about labeling AIDS as a disease of blacks or minorities. David Baltimore, cochairman of the National Academy of Sciences AIDS Commission, stated that candidates in the 1988 presidential elections could ignore AIDS because of the perception that AIDS would not affect the *general community,* "the phrase we are using to cover for the white, middle-class world" (Thomas, 1988, p. 56). Beny Primm, member of the Presidential Commission on AIDS, has said that the pressure to deal with AIDS may fall off as more cases occur in blacks and Hispanics: "The more 'ghettoization' of HIV infection and AIDS there is, the more rapidly research and treatment dollars will decrease" (Thomas, 1988, p. 56). And June Osborn, dean of the University of Michigan School of Public Health, has stated that, as

AIDS becomes overrepresented in the so-called underclass, "the most horrible scenario I can think of is that we decide 40,000 cases a year isn't so bad" (Thomas, 1988, p. 56).

To be sure, a lot of attention is being paid to the prevalence of AIDS in minorities. Almost every public pronouncement about the AIDS epidemic has addressed the special issue of AIDS in minorities. The U.S. surgeon general has addressed the issue; the Presidential Commission on AIDS devoted a section of its final report to the issue; and national conferences on AIDS in minorities have been held by the CDC in conjunction with other organizations. The conference of the Association of State and Territorial Health Officials held in Washington, D.C., in February 1988 was devoted almost entirely to the issue. And the U.S. Senate passed a bill in 1987 (S.B. 1872) "to provide for minority populations outreach, education, counseling, prevention, and research activities relating to acquired immune deficiency syndrome, and for other purposes." The bill provided for the appropriation of $30 million for fiscal year 1988, $35 million for fiscal year 1989, and $40 million for fiscal year 1990.

In addition to governmental activities, there are organizations such as the National Minority AIDS Council, Multicultural Inquiry and Research on AIDS, and many other local organizations devoted to the issue. The U.S. Conference of Mayors was awarded a grant by the CDC in 1987 to work with minority-oriented community-based organizations on AIDS education and prevention at the local level. Health care organizations such as the Institute of Medicine/National Academy of Sciences also have addressed the issue.

There is no question that something needs to be done about the very high rate of AIDS among minorities, and much is being done by various segments of the society. But the central question is why there is such a disproportionately high rate of AIDS in these populations. This question needs to be more adequately and comprehensively addressed before any effective control efforts—that is, prevention of further spread of AIDS in minorities—can succeed. While many researchers declare that the reason is not known, there has been a tendency to "blame" intravenous (IV) drug use for the trends.

However, of all blacks with AIDS, only 35% of men and 32% of women (average, 34%) were IV drug users. Obviously, the majority of black AIDS patients did not acquire the disease through IV drug use. Indeed, homosexual/bisexual behavior is the highest risk factor for AIDS in blacks (44%). More significantly, blacks have a disproportionately high rate of AIDS in all risk groups except hemophiliacs (CDC, 1990).

If IV drug use is not the primary reason for the disproportionately high rate, and if there is a similar rate in all risk groups, what other factors are there? As stated earlier, the role of genetics has been suggested. Though the scientific proof of the genetic basis has not been well established, several reports seem to suggest that something inherent in black people, genes or otherwise, makes them particularly susceptible to AIDS. A study reported in *The New England Journal of Medicine* in 1987 on the prevalence of human immunodeficiency virus (HIV) said in its abstract: "The following demographic factors were found to be *significant independent* predictors of positive HIV-antibody test; age, *black race*" [italics added] (Burke, 1987). Another report in the same journal in 1988 on the same topic stated: "HIV positivity was *independently* associated with increased age, *black race*" [italics added] (Quinn, 1988, p. 197).

The phrases *independent predictors of* and *independently associated with* imply that there is something specific about being black and the acquisition of AIDS. These kinds of phrases lend support to the gene theory, although the role of genes in the acquisition of AIDS is far from proved. I believe it is too early to "blame" the high rate of AIDS in blacks on genes just as it is inappropriate to do the same for IV drug use. There is a tendency to explain away—to rationalize—and do little else if answers are "found" too soon. I share Dr. Primm's concern about research and treatment dollar decreasing; I am also concerned that, if genetics were widely and prematurely accepted as the reason, further research could be slowed because of the mind-set that "we know why, but not much can be done about something they are born with."

Black people may have elevated levels of the Gc1F gene, but this does not explain—at least not entirely—the high rate of AIDS. I contend that the reason for its prevalence in black Americans and black Africans is more basic. It has to do with their overall health status. It has to do with the health care systems that serve them.

As stated earlier in this chapter, when I am asked why there is such a high rate of AIDS in blacks, my response is that it is not known exactly why. But I add that it has to do with the same reason that the rate of heart disease, stroke, diabetes, hypertension, cancer, tuberculosis, syphilis, and so on is higher in blacks than whites. Blacks are at a disadvantage in terms of the U.S. health care system; they tend to have less access to health care because of both physical and fiscal barriers. Consequently, they are less healthy overall than whites.

The acquisition of AIDS involves two major steps: transmission of the virus from an infected person to another person, and the development of immune system breakdown that leads to the diseases that constitute "AIDS." Both steps depend a lot on the general health of the individual before being exposed to the virus. There is evidence that preexisting conditions such as genital ulcers and certain viral illnesses promote both HIV transmission and progression to AIDS. Immune system integrity and function depend on coexisting illnesses, nutritional status, and, possibly, stress. Thus a person in generally poor health is more likely to develop AIDS once infected with the virus. Therefore, a plan to address the disproportionately high rate of AIDS in blacks should address the disproportionately high overall rate of other diseases. Plans aimed at correcting the alarming rates of AIDS in blacks should also aim at correcting the overall poor health of blacks.

The above discussion is what I had been "preaching" for the last several years. I was, therefore, delighted by a comment made by Admiral James Watkins, chairman of the Presidential Commission on AIDS, on June 1, 1988. On that day, he announced the completion of the commission's work and discussed some of the major recommendations. One of his comments on a television interview was that HIV has opened a window of opportunity to do something about the whole health care system, which puts certain segments of the population at a disadvantage.

I was delighted by Admiral Watkins's comment and the discussion of the issue in the commission's final report because a problem that has been ignored for so long might be receiving due attention. I have maintained for a long time that there is nothing mysterious about the disproportionately high rate of AIDS in blacks. Genes may play some role, but my contention is that environment—economic, social, cultural, and health environment—provides the overriding stimulus for the trend. The following chapters in the book represent my attempt to shed a little more light on a complex issue. I will provide epidemiological, basic scientific, and clinical evidence to explain my position. I will start with the general health status of blacks before discussing AIDS per se.

# REFERENCES

Burke, T. C., et al. (1987). Human immunodeficiency virus among civilian applicants for United States military service, October 1985 to March 1986. *The New England Journal of Medicine, 317,* 131-136.

Diager, S. P., & Brewton, C. S. (1987). Genetic susceptibility to AIDS: Absence of an association with group-specific component (Gc). *The New England Journal of Medicine, 317,* 631-632.

Eales, L. J., et al. (1987, May 2). Association of different allelic forms of group specific component with susceptibility to and clinical manifestation of human immunodeficiency virus infection. *Lancet,* pp. 999-1002.

Gilles, K., et al. (1987). Genetic susceptibility to AIDS: Absence of an association with group-specific component (Gc). *The New England Journal of Medicine, 317,* 630-631.

Harris County Medical Society and the Houston Academy of Medicine. (1987). *AIDS: A Guide for Survival.* Houston, TX: Author.

Institute of Medicine/National Academy of Sciences. (1988). *Confronting AIDS: Update 1988.* Washington, DC: National Academy Press.

Peterson, J., & Bakerman, R. (1988). The epidemiology of adult minority AIDS. *Multicultural Inquiry and Research on AIDS, 2,* 1-2.

Presidential Commission. (1988). *Report of the Presidential Commission on Human Immunodeficiency Virus Infection Epidemic.* Washington, DC: Author.

Quinn, T. C., et al. (1988). Human immunodeficiency virus infection among patients attending clinics for sexually transmitted diseases. *The New England Journal of Medicine, 318,* 197-202.

Quintanilla, A. (1987). *Genetically-controlled disease resistance and possible genetic markers for AIDS susceptibility.* San Francisco: Multicultural Inquiry and Research on AIDS.

Reports on selected racial/ethnic groups. (1988). *Morbidity and Mortality Weekly Report, 37,* 1-10.

Thomas, P. (1988, June 13). Press lets candidates off the hook on AIDS questions. *Medical World News,* p. 56.

U.S. Centers for Disease Control. (1990, October). *HIV/AIDS surveillance report.*

U.S. Senate, 100th congressional session. (1987, November 17). S. 1872. Minority Acquired Immunodeficiency Syndrome (AIDS) Awareness and Prevention Projects Act of 1987. Washington, DC.

# 2

# The Health Status of
# Black Americans

In 1984, then secretary of health and human services, Margaret Heckler, established the secretary's Task Force on Black and Minority Health. The task force was to investigate the disparity in morbidity and mortality rates experienced by blacks and other minorities in comparison with whites. This disparity had existed since accurate data on such matters had been kept by the federal government.

The task force issued a comprehensive report in 1985 (U.S. Department of Health and Human Services, 1985) detailing the clear differences between blacks and whites in terms of health status. It confirmed what had been known for decades—that blacks are less healthy, have higher mortality rates, and die at a younger age. Blacks have higher morbidity and mortality rates than whites in virtually every disease category, in every age group, and in both sexes. The report also confirmed that blacks are poorer, less educated, and less employed than whites. Recent reports indicate that things have not improved much for blacks and, in some cases, are worse. The 1985 report used data from the late 1970s and early 1980s, the period corresponding to the onset of the AIDS epidemic.

There is no question that a relationship exists between socioeconomic health and physical health. Black Americans have historically been less healthy socioeconomically than whites. The situation in the late 1970s and early 1980s was no different.

# SOCIOECONOMIC CHARACTERISTICS
# OF BLACKS

Data from 1980 show that blacks constituted 11.5% of the total U.S. population. This percentage was unevenly distributed by age group: at and under age 15, blacks constituted 15% of the total population, while they constituted only 8% by age 64. This clearly demonstrates that blacks die at an earlier age, shrinking their population after age 64. Of the total black population, females accounted for nearly 53%. Again, this was unevenly distributed. Under age 15 females accounted for 50% of the black population but over age 64 females accounted for 60%, indicating that black men die even earlier (U.S. Department of Health and Human Services, 1985).

About 59% of all blacks lived in inner-city areas of large cities, often in poor housing conditions. Overcrowding was a major problem. The average birth per woman for blacks was 2.3 compared with 1.7 for whites. About 38% of black households were headed by women, which was more than three times that of whites (about 11%). About 48% of first marriages among black women had been dissolved (separation, divorce, widowhood); the corresponding figure for white women was 30%. About 33% of black women who headed households had never been married. And more than 50% of black children lived in one-parent homes.

Compared with 87% of whites, only 79% of blacks had completed high school, and only 13% of blacks had completed college. The median income of black families was $15,430, which was about half that of white families. Among female-headed households, the median income for blacks was $8,650; it was $15,130 for white households. The percentage of blacks living below the poverty level (34%) was nearly three times that of whites (12%). Unemployment among blacks was nearly 16% compared with less than 7% for whites, and the rate for black teenagers was more than 40%. Black work force representation was primarily in nonskilled labor. Blacks constituted only 5% of all administrators, managers, and executives; 7% of professionals; 8% of technicians; 10% of clerical staff; 18% of service personnel; and 41% of private household personnel.

Utilization of health care by blacks was fragmented. Compared with 13% of whites, 20% of blacks had no usual source of medical care; 18% percent of blacks versus 9% of whites had no health insurance. A physician's office was reported as the usual source of care for 48% of blacks; it was 70% for whites. More than 25% of physician visits for blacks were in hospital clinics or emergency rooms, compared with 11% for whites.

The above socioeconomic data clearly demonstrate the bad state of affairs for blacks in comparison with whites. In many cases, blacks were worse off than other minorities. And there is nothing new about this phenomenon; this has been the history of blacks in the United States—before and after the secretary's Task Force on Black and Minority Health in 1985. Epidemiological studies throughout the world have clearly demonstrated the relation between the health status and the socioeconomic status of a population. The less educated, employed, and economically well off a group of people, the less healthy they are. Conversely, improvement in socioeconomic status results in improvement in health status. Therefore, it is not surprising that blacks have had such high mortality rates as presented at the beginning of this chapter. The suboptimal health status of average blacks starts at birth.

## INFANT HEALTH

It is clear from Table 2.1 that the greatest disparity in mortality rates between blacks and whites is with infant mortality. Blacks are more than twice as likely as whites to die in infancy. Infancy, as far as mortality rates are concerned, encompasses two periods: the neonatal period (from birth to 28 days of life) and the postneonatal period (from 28 days to one year of life). Neonatal mortality is more a reflection of the health status of the mother during pregnancy (and, many times, prior to pregnancy). Postneonatal death has more to do with living conditions and the quality of care the child receives. Neonatal deaths account for most of infant mortality in both blacks and whites. And blacks have higher mortality rates in both neonatal and postneonatal periods.

A major contributor to neonatal mortality is mothers' delivering low birth weight (LBW) babies, defined as a baby weighing less than

**Table 2.1**  Age-Adjusted Mortality Rates of Black and White Americans, 1980 (Rate Per 100,000 Population)

| Cause of Death | Black Male | White Male | Relative Risk | Black Female | White Female | Relative Risk |
|---|---|---|---|---|---|---|
| All causes | 1,112.8 | 745.3 | 1.5 | 631.1 | 411.1 | 1.5 |
| Heart disease | 327.3 | 277.5 | 1.2 | 201.1 | 134.6 | 1.5 |
| Cancer | 229.9 | 160.5 | 1.4 | 129.7 | 107.7 | 1.2 |
| Accident | 82.0 | 62.3 | 1.3 | 25.1 | 21.4 | 1.2 |
| Stroke | 77.5 | 41.9 | 1.9 | 61.7 | 35.2 | 1.8 |
| Homicide | 71.9 | 10.9 | 6.6 | 13.7 | 3.2 | 4.3 |
| Cirrhosis | 30.6 | 15.7 | 2.0 | 14.4 | 7.0 | 2.1 |
| Diabetes | 17.7 | 9.5 | 1.9 | 22.1 | 8.7 | 2.5 |
| Infant mortality | 2,586.7 | 1,230.3 | 2.1 | 2,123.7 | 962.5 | 2.2 |

SOURCE: Based on U.S. Department of Health and Human Services data.

2,500 grams (or about 5.5 pounds) at birth. LBW usually results from inadequate nutrient intake before and particularly during pregnancy. Black females are more likely to be pregnant as teenagers and out of wedlock. This type of mother has two potential problems: (a) She is still growing and requires more nutrient energy for her own growth and development, so she is not likely to transfer enough nutrients to the baby; (b) the typical black teenager who gets pregnant comes from a poor home, so her prepregnancy nutrient intake is likely to be suboptimal and is not likely to improve during pregnancy. Another major contributor to LBW is inadequate prenatal care. In 1983, 39% of black mothers did not receive any prenatal care in the first trimester compared with 21% of white mothers. Other contributing factors are cigarette smoking, illicit drug use, alcohol consumption, and frequent infections; these factors predominate in blacks.

The postnatal period obviously also has a lot to do with state of health at birth. A LBW child, if it survives the neonatal period, may still be in danger of not surviving the postneonatal period. A child whose nutrient intake is inadequate both in utero and after birth is susceptible to infections, particularly in a crowded environment. Other factors such as lack of immunization, maternal education, and general health affect postneonatal survival regardless of birth weight.

Infant health is influenced by many factors, both biological and environmental. Preexisting diseases of the mother, LBW at birth, congenital diseases, poor nutrition during pregnancy and after birth, crowded living situations, and lack of breast-feeding all influence infant health. All these factors depend a lot upon wealth and education. Blacks are less educated and less wealthy; they tend to possess more of the contributing factors. If a child born under such poor conditions survives infancy, it starts life at a disadvantage. Raised under such poor conditions, a child is likely to grow through adolescence to adulthood in poor health—both physical and socioeconomic health.

## CHILD AND ADOLESCENT HEALTH

More than for any other age group, the morbidity and mortality of children and adolescents are influenced by socioeconomic conditions. Major causes of illness and death in this age group are accidents, homicide, suicide, and substance abuse—all influenced by socioeconomic status. Another problem concerning adolescent health is teenage pregnancy; the rate is higher in lower socioeconomic groups.

Like black infants and adults, black children and adolescents are poorer and less educated than their white counterparts. In 1981, about 50% of blacks under 18 years of age lived below the poverty level compared with less than 15% of whites. Blacks under 18 had a higher rate of accidents, homicide, and substance abuse than whites, although whites had a higher rate of suicide than blacks. Substance abuse has a particularly devastating effect on a community. It carries with it a higher dropout rate from school as well as crime, prostitution, and several diseases. An IV drug user risks acquiring hepatitis and other infectious diseases in addition to the effect of the drug itself on the his or her body.

Teenage pregnancy has been a major problem in the black community. In 1981, 22% of black females had at least one baby by age 18; the corresponding figure for white females was 8%. Teenage mothers are more likely to be unmarried, to drop out of school, and to be dependent on welfare. Given that these mothers are poor and uneducated, they tend to receive less prenatal care, have inadequate nutrient intake, and thus have high rates of LBW deliveries. In addition to high infant mortality, teenagers have more complicated deliveries and high maternal mortality. In 1983, the maternal mortality rate for blacks was 18.3 per 100,000 population; it was 5.9 for whites.

## ADULT HEALTH

According to data from 1982, the life expectancy for blacks was 65 years for men and 74 years for women; it was 72 years and 79 years for white men and women, respectively. In 1980, the age-adjusted mortality rate for all causes was 1,112.8 per 100,000 population for black men, while it was 745.3 for white men; it was 631.1 and 411.1 for black women and white women, respectively. Blacks had higher mortality rates than whites in all eight leading causes of death (see Table 2.1).

A major finding of the secretary's Task Force on Black and Minority Health was the large number of *excess deaths* in blacks, which it defined as deaths that should not have occurred had blacks experienced the same age-sex death rates as whites. Between 1979 and 1981, there were an average of 59,000 excess deaths in blacks under age 70. This represented 42.3% of all deaths in blacks under age 70. Table 2.2 displays the leading cause of death for blacks in that time period. It shows excess deaths for blacks in every category.

The task force also defined *relative risk* as the ratio of the minority death rate to that of whites. This accounts for differences in population size. In 1980, the relative risk for blacks of death from all causes was 1.96 for males and 1.93 for females. This means that a black

**Table 2.2**  Average Annual Number of Deaths of Blacks Under Age 70, 1979-1981

| Cause of Death | Males | | | Females | | |
|---|---|---|---|---|---|---|
| | Observed | Expected | Excess | Observed | Expected | Excess |
| Cardiovascular disease | 24,913 | 16,444 | 8,469 | 17,788 | 8,076 | 9,712 |
| Cancer | 16,117 | 10,335 | 5,782 | 11,946 | 9,677 | 2,269 |
| Cirrhosis | 2,706 | 1,344 | 1,362 | 1,525 | 743 | 782 |
| Infant mortality | 6,782 | 3,465 | 3,317 | 5,540 | 2,679 | 2,861 |
| Diabetes | 1,190 | 544 | 646 | 1,786 | 583 | 1,203 |
| Accidents | 8,429 | 7,316 | 1,113 | 2,739 | 2,605 | 134 |
| Homicide | 7,935 | 1,227 | 6,708 | 1,796 | 415 | 1,381 |
| All others | 16,629 | 8,914 | 7,715 | 10,817 | 5,614 | 5,203 |
| Total deaths | 84,701 | 49,589 | 35,112 | 53,937 | 30,392 | 23,545 |

SOURCE: Based on U.S. Department of Health and Human Services data.

person in 1980 was twice as likely to die from all causes as a white person. As evident in Table 2.1, blacks had high relative risk in all eight leading causes of death. In addition, blacks were 16.5 times more likely to die from tuberculosis, 11.8 times from hypertension, and 5.6 times from anemias.

Why the high rate for excess deaths in blacks? Why the high relative risk? Are these trends dependent upon or related to genetics? Again, I maintain that genes may or may not play a role, but the overriding factor is the total environment. Analysis of selected health conditions should shed further light on the issue.

## Heart Disease

Heart disease is and has been the leading cause of death for all Americans since the 1950s. It is also the leading cause of death for blacks. As shown in both Tables 2.1 and 2.2, the heart disease death rate is higher for blacks than for whites. The death rate from heart disease has been decreasing for all Americans since 1968, but recent studies have demonstrated that the rate of decrease has slowed down for blacks since 1976 (U.S. Department of Health and Human Services, 1985).

The three major risk factors for heart disease are high serum cholesterol, hypertension, and cigarette smoking. Other contributors are family history, diabetes, being overweight, and physical inactivity. All of these risk factors are more prevalent in blacks. Blacks tend to eat foods high in cholesterol and saturated fats. They tend to be less involved in smoking cessation programs, and tobacco company advertising is selectively targeted toward minorities and the poor. Blacks also tend to get hypertension at an earlier age and treat it less.

All these risk factors are influenced by the social environment, which is related to heart disease mortality; mortality is related to income, education, and employment. The decline in heart disease mortality mentioned above was more prominent in areas with the highest income, education, and white-collar employment. Studies in Great Britain have shown that heart disease mortality is higher in the lower classes. Also between 1970 and 1980, there was a decline in heart disease mortality among British nonmanual workers but not in manual workers.

If the prevalence of all risk factors for heart disease is higher in blacks; if social environment influences heart disease mortality; and if blacks are less educated, less employed, and less wealthy—it should not be surprising that the mortality rate is higher for blacks, and it should not be surprising that the decline in heart disease mortality is less steep for blacks.

## Stroke

Mortality from stroke has been higher in blacks than whites, though mortality has declined for all races since the 1960s. In addition, of those who survive a stroke, blacks tend to have more severe and permanent disabilities.

Strokes are often divided into two causal groups—"cholesterol stroke" and "hypertension stroke." The so-called cholesterol stroke results from a blood clot in one or more brain vessels. When a clot breaks off from a cholesterol plaque in the heart or major artery and blocks a vessel in the brain, the brain tissue beyond the blockage may die, resulting in a stroke. If the blocked vessel did not supply a large area, death may not result, and disability may be less severe. The "hypertension stroke" results from bleeding into brain tissue, often a result of hypertension. In the presence of uncontrolled hypertension, the very high pressure used to pump blood may rupture a brain vessel or vessels. Again, death or the degree of disability depends upon how much brain tissue dies from the bleed.

Hypertension strokes tend to affect a wider area of brain tissue and thus cause more death and disability than cholesterol strokes. Obviously, there is an interaction between cholesterol plaques and hypertension. In any case, it is clear that blacks have a higher prevalence of hypertension, and strokes in blacks tend to be of the hypertension type. Hypertension also is related to social environment as will be discussed later.

## Cancer

It is often said that the word *cancer* is a misnomer; that is, there are many types of cancers: lung cancer, breast cancer, stomach cancer, and so on. All cancers as a group have been the second leading cause of death in the United States. Blacks have the highest cancer rates, both in incidence and in mortality, of all racial groups in the United States.

It is estimated that about 30% of cancer is related to cigarette smoking, 35% is related to diet, and 3% is related to alcohol intake. Cigarette smoking is related to cancer of the lung, throat, pancreas, and urinary bladder. High-fat diet is related to cancer of the breast, colon, prostate, and uterus; high-fiber diet is associated with low incidence of breast and colon cancer. Alcohol is related to cancer of the mouth, larynx, esophagus, and liver.

As stated before, there are more black smokers than smokers in other racial groups. Blacks tend to have high-fat diets. And, although there is no clear-cut evidence that blacks consume more alcohol, the higher prevalence of cirrhosis indicates relatively high alcohol consumption by blacks. Studies have shown that socioeconomic status is a major contributing factor both in incidence of and in surviving cancer. Socioeconomic status affects the use of cigarettes, alcohol, and diet. It thus contributes to the very high incidence and mortality rates for cancer in blacks.

## Hypertension

Hypertension, or high blood pressure, is the leading morbid condition in blacks. The rate of hypertension is higher in blacks than in all other racial groups for all age groups and for both sexes. Blacks suffer more frequently from end-organ damage (heart disease, stroke, kidney failure) and mortality secondary to hypertension. Hypertension in blacks tends to be salt dependent and is better managed by restricting salt intake. Also, black hypertensives often have low serum potassium and calcium. These characteristics have led to the suggestion that there is a genetic basis to the disease. But there are prevalence differences among black populations in different geographic areas, suggesting environmental factors. The prevalence of hypertension is higher in black Americans than blacks in the Caribbean, and the prevalence in Caribbean blacks is higher than in African blacks. In the United States, the prevalence is lower in blacks of higher socioeconomic status; the opposite prevails in African blacks. In an earlier publication (Duh & Willingham, 1986), I suggested that these differences confirm studies suggesting that environmental stress is a major determinant of hypertension. This is particularly evident when one considers the way typical black Africans and black Americans respond to stress.

The dominant U.S. culture emphasizes competition, individual achievement, and equal opportunity. The notion of equal opportunity and availability of resources implies that, if one tries hard enough, one will succeed. Having been subjected to all kinds of discrimination, many blacks have had to try harder; they are subjected to stress earlier in life and sustain it longer. Furthermore, many poor blacks live in crowded, high-tension neighborhoods—a huge source of stress. Blacks of high socioeconomic status do not have to face the pressure of poverty and the need to rise above it.

In many black African societies, emphasis is on communal accomplishment, with the extended family system functioning as the backbone of the community. Black Africans of lower socioeconomic status often seek help from relatives or even neighbors and thus deal with stress in a passive manner. The well-educated city-dwelling Africans of higher socioeconomic status tend to encounter stress "Western style" as well as from traditional sources. The nature of education and city dwelling bring about a level of competition and individual accomplishment with some traditional tensions. In addition, the extended family system makes such individuals *superfathers,* that is, in addition to their own nuclear families, other less affluent relatives approach them with all kinds of problems—a huge source of stress.

Genetics may play a role in the pathogenesis of hypertension, but both laboratory and epidemiological evidence has demonstrated the predominant contribution of stress. The differences in prevalence between U.S. and African blacks as discussed above confirm the importance of stress. Like every other condition so far discussed, hypertension in black Americans has a lot to do with low socioeconomic status.

## Diabetes

Diabetes is another major cause of death that is more prevalent in blacks than whites; in 1980, the prevalence in blacks was twice that in whites. Diabetes also contributes to other diseases such as heart disease and peripheral vascular disease.

There are two major types of diabetes—insulin-dependent diabetes mellitus (IDDM) and noninsulin-dependent diabetes mellitus (NIDDM). IDDM usually occurs in children and young adults; NIDDM usually occurs in middle-aged and older adults. The NIDDM type accounts for 90% to 95% of the disease; it is commonly associated with obesity, and it is the type that affects blacks more than whites. Diabetes is a dangerous disease because of the many body organs it affects. It causes heart disease, blindness, kidney failure, and vascular complications, which often lead to amputation.

The role of obesity—fat accumulation in the body—in NIDDM is quite well established. Fat interferes with both insulin secretion by the pancreas and cell uptake and utilization of insulin. Therefore, medications to treat NIDDM are often not very effective in obese individuals. The best way to control diabetes and prevent its complications is to combine medication with a carefully devised diet.

Blacks die more frequently from diabetes and suffer more complications from the disease because of inadequate care. They tend to be more obese, to be poorer, and to seek medical care later in the disease process, and they are less likely to follow physician instructions fully. Many physicians do not take time to explain well the disease process and the role of medication, diet, and exercise. They often do not develop individualized meal plans; they simply tell patients to take the medicine properly, eat the right foods, and exercise. There is epidemiological evidence that poor blacks often do not understand their doctor's instructions and are reluctant to ask questions, especially when the doctor is white.

**Tuberculosis**

As stated earlier, the relative risk of tuberculosis (TB) for blacks in comparison with whites was 16.5 in 1980. Few diseases are influenced more by socioeconomic status than TB. Studies from throughout the world have clearly demonstrated a higher prevalence of TB among populations that are poor and live under crowded conditions. Because of the efficiency of transmission under crowded conditions, TB is quite common in refugee camps, prisons, shelters, and poorly run day-care centers.

Tuberculosis is transmitted through the air. When patients with pulmonary TB cough, sneeze, speak, or sing, the infectious agent of the disease is released into the air. Obviously, the efficiency with which the released particles enter another person's body depends upon how close the contact is. Once the particles are inhaled by a susceptible host, the host's immune system tries to contain the infection. Usually the organism remains trapped in the body without the development of clinical manifestations and potential for transmission to others. If the host's immune system does not function optimally, the disease process may progress. Sometimes, the trapped organisms are reactivated after many years if immune status changes or in the presence of other illnesses such as diabetes.

In light of the infectious process, TB is more likely to occur in children under 5 years, whose immune systems are not fully developed, and in older people, whose immune status is decreased due to the aging process. Other susceptible people include those on immuno-suppressive medications, alcoholics, the homeless, IV drug users, and those with poor nutrition and high stress. It is apparent, then, why blacks have such a high rate of TB. It is important to note that the rate is highest in poor blacks. Crowded housing conditions, poor nutrition, high levels of stress, IV drug use, and the presence of other illnesses provide for both efficient transmission and development of tuberculosis.

## Sexually Transmitted Diseases

For many decades, efforts by public health officials to control sexually transmitted diseases (STDs) were mainly focused on gonorrhea and syphilis. However, many more STDs—*Chlamydia trachomatis,* genital herpes, hepatitis, and genital warts—were recognized as major health problems in the 1970s. The prevalence of these "newer" STDs, particularly chlamydia and genital herpes, exceeds that of gonorrhea and syphilis. All the STDs combined produce a host of diseases and complications and cost billions of dollars.

In addition to such symptoms as burning, itching, discharge, and ulcers manifested during the acute phases of STDs, major complications occur with untreated or inadequately treated STDs. For example, pelvic inflammatory disease (PID) is estimated to cause involuntary infertility in 200,000 U.S. women yearly. An estimated 336,600 infants are born to mothers with chlamydial infections—pneumonia and conjunctivitis. Genital herpes may cause miscarriages, stillbirth, or severe neurological damage to infants.

Whether complications result from STDs depends upon whether the infected person is treated, when during the disease process treatment is instituted, and how adequate the treatment is. There are several potential problems with the treatment of STDs: (a) There is a very high rate of asymptomatic infections—the carrier may not be aware of the infection and thus may not seek treatment. (b) Very accurate and inexpensive diagnostic tests do not exist for many of the STDs. (c) Many people are embarrassed to discuss an illness involving sexual matters and often delay seeking treatment, hoping it will go away.

(d) Many doctors are not experienced in diagnosing, treating, and offering counseling to STD patients.

Blacks have a higher rate of STDs, and socioeconomic status is the main reason. Many poor blacks get treated for STDs at local health departments. These are usually overcrowded clinics where patients spend hours in waiting areas. There often is a lot of paperwork before a patient is seen. Some clinics see patients by appointment only. Some require a fee up front before a patient is seen. All these barriers often lead to delays in obtaining treatment. An important part of treatment is adequate counseling. The patient should understand the disease process so as to comply fully with treatment and return for follow-up. As mentioned earlier, poor blacks tend not to understand doctor's instructions. Also, because of the very high asymptomatic rates, many STDs are diagnosed and treated during routine or other visits to the doctor. Poor blacks do not see doctors often, and STDs are usually diagnosed during (late) symptomatic stages.

## Health Promotion/Disease Prevention

Health promotion and disease prevention involve activities in which individuals and society participate to reduce the burden of disease. Health promotion implies that an individual is healthy and doing certain things to be even healthier; weight control, smoking cessation, and stress management are examples of health promotion activities. Disease prevention may be practiced by a totally healthy person or by one who is not so healthy. There are three levels of prevention. *Primary prevention* involves activities to avoid the occurrence of an illness, such as vaccination against measles. *Secondary prevention* seeks to avoid complication from an illness, such as controlling blood pressure to avoid a stroke. *Tertiary prevention* attempts to preclude disability from disease or injury, such as physical therapy to avoid paralysis from a stroke.

Black Americans, particularly the inner-city poor, are much less likely to be involved in health promotion activities. As such, they have a higher prevalence of obesity and cigarette smoking as well as high levels of stress. They are less likely to eat healthful foods, to exercise, and to complete recommended immunizations. They are less likely to see a doctor for checkups and follow doctors' instructions on good health practices. All of these are based on poverty and lack of education.

In a 1988 conference in Atlanta on the promotion of the health of black Americans, experts concluded that information on nutrition and exercise is not reaching inner-city blacks. They eat a lot of so-called soul food, which is heavily laden with fat. Many of them do not have money to join health clubs. And high crime rates in some communities discourage such activities as walking on the streets or in parks. It was concluded that poor nutrition and lack of exercise are responsible for the poor health of many blacks.

It should be obvious to the reader from the discussion in this chapter that black Americans on the average are less healthy than other racial groups. They have relatively lower life expectancy. They have higher mortality rates. Infant health, child and adolescent health, and adult health are all relatively poorer for them. They have high excess death rates and high relative risk rates for most health conditions. They are less likely to be involved in health promotion and disease prevention activities.

Black Americans are on the average also poorer. They are less educated and less employed. Many poor blacks live in crowded housing conditions, where crime, illicit drug use, and prostitution are common. They tend to be uninsured or underinsured. They tend to see doctors less often; they tend to wait until later stages of an illness before seeing a doctor. They tend to use public clinics or hospital emergency rooms instead of doctors' offices.

Black Americans are less healthy because of their lower socioeconomic status. As discussed in the chapter, every poor health conditions is related to low socioeconomic status. Blacks have both physical and fiscal barriers to health care. Dr. Quentin Young gave an example of these barriers at the 69th Annual Session of the American College of Physicians in New York City: New medical patients might wait for nine months to be seen in the outpatient clinics at the Cook County (Chicago) Hospital (Snyder, 1988).

The dual poor health and low socioeconomic status of blacks have been present for generations. In the late 1970s and early 1980s, blacks were poorer and less healthy. In the late 1980s, they were as poor or even poorer than they were before. In the late 1970s and early 1980s, when AIDS was emerging as a disease, it makes sense that AIDS would affect people who were less healthy already. The connection between poor health and the acquisition of AIDS will be clearer in the next few chapters.

# REFERENCES

Duh, S. V., & Willingham, D. F. (1986). An ecological view of hypertension in blacks. *Journal of the National Medical Association, 78,* 617-619.

Sellers, T. (1988). Fitness and diet needs unmet for innercity residents. *Urban Medicine, 3,* 12-17.

Semples, G., et al. (1988). Divergence of the recent trends in coronary mortality for the four major race-sex-groups. *American Journal of Public Health, 78,* 1422-1427.

Snyder, F. (1988). Inner-city citizens are often uninsured and underserved. *Urban Medicine, 3,* 14-18.

U.S. Department of Health Education and Welfare. (1979). *Healthy people: The surgeon general's report on health promotion and disease prevention* (DHEW Publication No. 79-55071). Washington, DC: Government Printing Office.

U.S. Department of Health and Human Services. (1985). *Report of the Secretary's Task Force on Black and Minority Health: Vol 1. Executive summary.* Washington, DC: Government Printing Office.

U.S. Department of Health and Human Services. (1988). *Disease prevention/health promotion: The facts.* Palo Alto, CA: Bull.

White-Clergerie, A. (1988). Racial differences in cerebrovascular disease. *Urban Medicine, 3,* 8-9.

Wing, S. (1988). Social inequalities in the decline of coronary mortality. *American Journal of Public Health, 78,* 1415-1416.

# 3

# History and Epidemiology of AIDS

It has been said that organized medicine's most significant accomplishment has been the conquest of infectious disease, at least in the developed countries. At the turn of the century, infectious diseases such as tuberculosis and pneumonia caused most of the deaths worldwide. Syphilis and leprosy were major causes of illness. Viral illnesses such as polio and measles killed millions. And we remember the bubonic plague epidemic, which killed millions in Europe. The development of powerful antibiotics and vaccines afforded the control of these killer diseases; and, in the case of smallpox, total eradication has occurred.

Infectious disease was conquered mainly because of improvement in environmental and personal hygiene influenced by improvement in socioeconomic status. This, of course, is why the phenomenon is more prominent in the developed nations. Infectious disease as a killer was replaced by the so-called diseases of civilization—heart disease, cancer, stroke, and so on. Most research efforts in the past several decades had been focused on the new killer diseases, and scientists were basically "sleeping" in terms of infectious disease. Then, suddenly, they were awakened in the early 1980s by a killer infectious disease—acquired immunodeficiency syndrome (AIDS). This disease is communicable; it kills rather quickly; and there is no cure or effective treatment.

In 1980, physicians started seeing patients in different parts of the United States with similar but unusual presentations. They were basically young men who previously had been healthy who were afflicted with unusual illnesses. These were diseases that had not caused any significant illnesses previously, but these young men were very ill. More important, their illnesses did not respond to usual therapy, and the patients died. They suffered mainly from *Pneumocystis carinii* pneumonia (PCP), a rare lung infection, and Kaposi's sarcoma, a normally benign cancer.

The first few cases were reported by physicians in Los Angeles and New York. In June and July 1981, five cases of PCP from Los Angeles and 26 cases of Kaposi's sarcoma from New York and Los Angeles were reported to the Centers for Disease Control (CDC). All these were in male homosexuals. By 1982, AIDS was being recognized in IV drug users and Haitians. It was being found in recipients of blood or blood products, infants, heterosexual partners of AIDS patients, and Africans by early 1983. Subsequently, it became apparent that anyone could acquire the disease anywhere in the world. By the middle of 1988, 175 countries were reporting AIDS to the World Health Organization (WHO). It truly had become pandemic.

Initially, AIDS was an enigma. It was not known what caused it, how it was transmitted, and why the victims all died. It did not take scientists too long to unravel the mystery. First, it became clear that something was destroying the victims' immune systems and leaving them vulnerable to unusual diseases. Then the routes of transmission became fairly clear. The establishment of probable routes of transmission led to the suggestion that the cause might be an infectious agent or agents. Some scientists suggested a combination of infectious diseases; others suggested a single agent. Meanwhile, scientists were busy trying to find the cause(s). By 1982, a case definition had been developed for reporting purposes though it was not known what caused the disease.

A single agent was identified in 1983 as the cause of AIDS simultaneously by scientists in France and the United States. Both teams isolated a single virus from a number of AIDS patients. The French team, headed by Dr. Luc Montagnier, named the virus *lymphadenopathy-associated virus* (LAV). Dr. Robert Gallo and his team at the U.S. National Cancer Institute named it *human T-cell lymphotrophic virus III* (HTLV-III). The virus was referred to in the scientific milieu as HTLV-III/LAV to satisfy both sets of scientists. In 1986, an international nomenclature committee sought to simplify matters by naming the virus *human immunodeficiency virus* (HIV).

The discovery of HIV was a huge step in the understanding and possible control of AIDS. By 1984, the virus had been recovered from a significant number of patients, and antibodies to the virus were found in both patients and nonpatients from populations at increased risk for AIDS. The detection of antibodies to HIV led to the control of one route of transmission—transfusion of blood or blood products. In June 1985, a laboratory test was licensed to screen blood for HIV antibodies. The enzyme-linked immunosorbent assay (ELISA) test is a serologic, or test-tube, test for quick screening. The Western Blot, which involves a more elaborate electrophoresis technique, is used to confirm a positive ELISA test. Both tests are used for diagnosing HIV infection and for screening donated blood. Since June 1985, all blood donated in the United States and many other countries has been screened for HIV antibodies. Though the tests are not 100% effective, it is quite safe to receive donated blood because all blood that tests positive is discarded; there is only about a 1 in 40,000 chance of acquiring AIDS through blood transfusion in the United States.

HIV has been very well studied and its chemical structure is well known. It is a retrovirus, meaning that, unlike other viruses that are made of RNA molecules, it contains an enzyme called *reverse transcriptase*, which allows it to reproduce itself. Like other retroviruses, it uses the infected person's cells to reproduce itself. By so doing, it kills these cells. The devastating effect of HIV is that it uses the person's T-lymphocytes, the type of white blood cells that help fight off infections. When enough of these lymphocytes are destroyed, the person develops AIDS.

Both the chemical structure of HIV and the place at which it attaches on the lymphocyte have been studied in an attempt to find a cure for AIDS. Much has been revealed but so far no cure has been discovered. Only one medicine, Retrovir (formerly AZT) had been approved for the treatment of AIDS by fall 1990. Retrovir inhibits reverse transcriptase to prevent the reproduction of HIV. Theoretically, therefore, it should cure AIDS, but, though most patients live longer while taking it, it has many serious side effects. And the patients ultimately die. Research continues, and scientists are working on many different drugs. Meanwhile, some unscrupulous people have distributed all kinds of quack therapies for AIDS.

A second approach to the control of AIDS is the development of a vaccine. Again, much work is being done by scientists all over the world, but a vaccine has not yet been developed. The major problem involving the development of a vaccine for HIV is the fact that the virus is so dangerous. The most effective and long-lasting vaccine is from the whole organism, alive or killed. But because HIV causes such a devastating disease as AIDS, scientists have been reluctant to discuss the whole-virus vaccine for HIV. Dr. Jonas Salk, who created the polio vaccine, is the only prominent scientist to advocate the whole-vaccine approach, but he has not received a lot of support from other scientists. Most of research effort has, therefore, been focused on isolating portions of the virus for vaccine development.

Various groups in the United States and other countries are at different stages of developing and testing a vaccine. In 1987, a French scientist, Daniel Sagury, injected himself with an experimental vaccine. A year later, he had not developed any ill effects. Most of the testing, however, has been done in volunteers with AIDS or HIV infection in the United States and Africa. During an international conference on AIDS in Africa in Tanzania in October 1988, Robert Gallo of the National Cancer Institute appealed to the Tanzanian health minister to permit large-scale trials of vaccines in Tanzania and other central African countries, but officials from those African countries did not embrace the idea.

*     *     *

One of the main reasons for the lack of cure and vaccine is the fact that there are many different strains of HIV and different types of viruses causing AIDS. In 1985, Dr. Myron Essex and his colleagues at the Harvard School of Public Health isolated a retrovirus from prostitutes and surgical patients in Senegal. They isolated the same virus from healthy individuals of that West African country in 1986. Also in 1986, Montagnier of the Institute Pasteur and his team isolated a retrovirus from two West Africans with AIDS in Lisbon, Portugal, and Paris, France. The virus isolated by both the Essex and the Montagnier teams was immunologically different than HIV. However, this virus seemed to be the cause of the AIDS in the two Montagnier patients. Subsequently, that virus was identified as the cause of AIDS in many patients; it has been designated HIV-2.

HIV-2 appears to be relatively common in West African countries and quite rare in countries in other parts of Africa. A few cases of HIV-2 AIDS have been found in Europe. In the United States, only one case of HIV-2 has been reported, in February 1988 in New Jersey. The virus was isolated from a patient with AIDS who had emigrated from West Africa. Significantly, the patient had developed the AIDS symptoms in the home country before going to the United States, implying that the virus was acquired there.

In July 1988, Dr. Guido van der Groen of the Institute of Tropical Medicine in Antwerp, Belgium, isolated yet another retrovirus from a man and his wife in Cameroon in West Africa. This new virus has been designated HIV-3. So, it appears that different retroviruses in addition to HIV-1 exist in West Africa. It is entirely possible that new viruses could be found in different populations, making the search for a cure and a vaccine for AIDS even more difficult.

For many years, there has been consensus that the only weapon available to fight AIDS is education. Because the transmission of HIV involves mostly personal behavior, AIDS is potentially fully preventable. Everybody needs to be educated about the disease so individual choices may be made to avoid the transmission of the virus. Yet, except in a few cases, education has not produced the expected results. Both educational programs and people's acceptance of messages have been less than adequate. Governmental and other agencies have not given the financial support needed for effective education. In some cases, there is not enough personnel to carry out programs. And the two major risk behaviors—IV drug use and sexual habits— are difficult to break.

Throughout the history of AIDS, there has been a lot of excitement and a lot of frustration. In the short period during which the disease has been identified, an incredible amount of knowledge has been acquired on all of its aspects, which has generated a lot of excitement in the scientific world. There has been an annual international conference on AIDS since 1985, during which a great deal of information is exchanged. At the end of the fourth conference in Stockholm, Sweden, in 1988, the venues for the next six years were announced. Despite the knowledge and excitement, there is still no cure or effective treatment; there is no vaccine; and educational programs have only been marginally effective. The pandemic continues, and the epidemiology of the disease has been fairly stable.

By the end of August 1990, a total of 283,010 cases of AIDS had been reported to WHO from 157 countries. The figure represents the cumulative total since 1981. The figure is widely believed to be only a fraction of actual cases because of underreporting, particularly in developing countries. The WHO estimates as many as 600,000 cases worldwide. The majority of cases (170,661) have been reported from the Americas, and Southeast Asia has reported the fewest number of

**Table 3.1**   Number of Reported AIDS Cases From Different Regions of the
World, as of August 31, 1990

| Region | Number of Cases | Number of Countries Reporting |
|---|---|---|
| Africa | 70,724 | 45 |
| Americas | 170,661 | 44 |
| Eastern Mediterranean | 481 | 16 |
| Europe | 38,503 | 31 |
| South East Asia | 107 | 5 |
| Western Pacific | 2,534 | 16 |
| Total | 283,010 | 157 |

SOURCE: Based on World Health Organization data.

cases (107). Table 3.1 displays the distribution of reported AIDS
cases in different regions of the world. There are relatively few means
of acquiring HIV—sexual intercourse, sharing IV drug needles, transfusion of blood and blood products, and from mother to infant
through birth.

In the Americas and Europe, homosexual activity and IV drug use
are the major means of acquisition. Transfusion represents only a
small proportion. In Africa, homosexual activity and IV drug use are
unusual and contribute very little to the acquisition of AIDS. The majority of AIDS cases there are acquired through heterosexual activity.
Because of logistic and other technical reasons, donated blood is not
as effectively screened for HIV, and blood transfusion is still a significant means of transmission. In addition, the use of unsterile needles
by health professionals in many African countries is a factor in the
transmission process.

In the United States, 143,746 cases of AIDS had been reported to
the CDC by the end of August 1990. The number of reported cases
doubled every six months to a year from 1981 through 1984. The dou-
bling has not occurred since 1985, but reported cases continue to increase consistently from year to year. Table 3.2 displays the number
of reported cases by year. The epidemiology of AIDS cases has been
changing in terms of means of transmission. The majority (69.9) were
through homosexual/bisexual activity through 1988, followed by IV
drug use (18%); heterosexual activity and transfusion of blood/blood
products contributed to relatively fewer cases. By September 1990,

**Table 3.2** Reported AIDS Cases and Case-Fatality Rates, United States, by Year

| Year | Cases | Deaths | Case-Fatality Rate |
|------|-------|--------|--------------------|
| 1981 | 291 | 255 | 91.8 |
| 1982 | 1,030 | 926 | 89.9 |
| 1983 | 2,838 | 2,573 | 90.6 |
| 1984 | 5,763 | 4,957 | 86.0 |
| 1985 | 10,628 | 8,892 | 83.7 |
| 1986 | 17,050 | 12,517 | 73.4 |
| 1987 | 24,082 | 12,829 | 53.3 |
| 1988 | 23,941 | 6,775 | 28.3 |

SOURCE: Based on U.S. Centers for Disease Control data.

homosexual activity contributed to 60% and IV drug use contributed to 22% of cases. There is an indication that heterosexual transmission is increasing at a faster rate.

In terms of racial groups in the United States, most AIDS cases (55%) have occurred in whites, but blacks and Hispanics are disproportionately represented in reported cases. Blacks constitute 28% of AIDS cases but constitute only 12% of the U.S. population. Hispanics constitute 16% of AIDS cases but represent 6% of the U.S. population. Furthermore, blacks and Hispanics account for 83% of cases in heterosexual men, 72% of cases in women, and 77% of cases in children. Of all U.S. cases associated with IV drug use, 48% have occurred in blacks and 32% in Hispanics. Of female AIDS cases, the proportion who were IV drug users was 57% for blacks and 51% for Hispanics; it was 40% for whites. Table 3.3 displays transmission categories and the racial distribution of AIDS cases. It is obvious from the table that blacks and Hispanics lead in every transmission category except that of hemophiliacs.

As large as the number of AIDS cases is, a bigger problem is the number of people with asymptomatic HIV infection. The CDC has estimated that between 1 and 1.5 million individuals in the United States may be infected with HIV. Worldwide, the estimate is 5 to 10 million. It is not known how many of those carrying the virus will develop AIDS. The CDC projects that 20% to 30% of the estimated number of HIV carriers will develop AIDS by 1991. A study in San Francisco projected that 35% will develop AIDS in 7 to 8 years and 50% in 10

**Table 3.3** The Distribution of AIDS Cases by Race/Ethnic Group and Transmission Category, United States, as of September 30, 1990

| Exposure Category | White, not Hispanic # | % | Black, not Hispanic # | % | Hispanic # | % | Asian/ Pacific Islander # | % | American Indian/ Alaska Native # | % | Total # | % |
|---|---|---|---|---|---|---|---|---|---|---|---|---|
| *Adult males* | | | | | | | | | | | | |
| Homosexual/bisexual contact | 63,669 | (80) | 15,043 | (44) | 9,445 | (46) | 692 | (81) | 116 | (63) | 89,155 | (66) |
| Intravenous (IV) drug use (heterosexual) | 5,004 | (6) | 11,884 | (35) | 7,882 | (39) | 26 | (3) | 20 | (11) | 24,890 | (18) |
| Homosexual/bisexual contact and IV drug use | 5,848 | (7) | 2,713 | (7) | 1,437 | (7) | 19 | (2) | 28 | (15) | 10,058 | (7) |
| Hemophilia/coagulation disorder | 1,078 | (1) | 82 | (0) | 101 | (1) | 19 | (2) | 8 | (4) | 1,289 | (1) |
| Heterosexual contact | 327 | (1) | 2,311 | (7) | 284 | (1) | 7 | (1) | 2 | (1) | 3,134 | (2) |
| Receipt of blood/blood products | 1,596 | (2) | 314 | (1) | 184 | (1) | 44 | (5) | 1 | (1) | 2,149 | (2) |
| Other undetermined | 1,731 | (2) | 1,522 | (4) | 1,015 | (5) | 50 | (6) | 9 | (5) | 4,371 | (3) |
| Male subtotal | 79,451 | (100) | 33,869 | (100) | 20,348 | (100) | 854 | (100) | 184 | (100) | 135,046 | (100) |
| *Adult females* | | | | | | | | | | | | |
| IV drug use | 1,537 | (40) | 4,296 | (57) | 1,493 | (51) | 13 | (17) | 16 | (55) | 7,367 | (51) |
| Hemophilia/coagulation disorder | 28 | (1) | 5 | (0) | 1 | (0) | — | — | — | — | 34 | (0) |
| Heterosexual contact | 1,127 | (29) | 2,401 | (32) | 1,073 | (37) | 27 | (35) | 8 | (28) | 4,651 | (32) |
| Receipt of blood/blood products | 884 | (23) | 274 | (4) | 173 | (6) | 26 | (34) | 2 | (7) | 1,363 | (9) |
| Other/undetermined | 278 | (7) | 558 | (7) | 180 | (6) | 11 | (14) | 3 | (10) | 1,037 | (7) |
| Female subtotal | 3,854 | (100) | 7,537 | (100) | 2,290 | (100) | 77 | (100) | 29 | (100) | 14,452 | (100) |
| Total for males and females | 83,305 | | 41,406 | | 23,268 | | 931 | | 213 | | 149,498 | |
| *Pediatric (less than 13 years old)* | | | | | | | | | | | | |
| Hemophilia/coagulation disorder | 89 | (16) | 17 | (1) | 23 | (3) | 3 | (25) | — | — | 132 | (5) |
| Mother with risk of HIV infection | 338 | (60) | 1,246 | (92) | 582 | (85) | 4 | (33) | 5 | (100) | 2,184 | (83) |
| Receipt of blood/blood products | 129 | (23) | 53 | (4) | 56 | (8) | 5 | (42) | — | — | 243 | (9) |
| Undetermined | 9 | (2) | 37 | (3) | 23 | (3) | — | — | — | — | 69 | (3) |
| Pediatric subtotal | 565 | (100) | 1,355 | (100) | 684 | (100) | 12 | (100) | 5 | (100) | 2,628 | (100) |
| Grand total | 83,870 | | 42,761 | | 23,952 | | 943 | | 218 | | 152,126 | |

SOURCE: Based on Centers for Disease Control data.

years. However, a San Francisco epidemiologist, Dr. George Lemp, more recently predicted that 100% of HIV carriers will develop AIDS in 16 years. Obviously, with these kind of projections, AIDS is going to continue to be a devastating problem in the future without a cure. And, as with AIDS cases, studies have shown a disproportionately higher prevalence of HIV infection in blacks and Hispanics than whites.

Several studies have been conducted nationwide on seroprevalence of HIV in different population groups. These have included military recruits, job corps applicants, clients attending sexually transmitted disease clinics, sentinel hospital patients, and blood donors. The studies have consistently shown that blacks and Hispanics have higher seropositivity rates than whites. Excess seropositivity in blacks over whites ranges from 2 to 15 in these studies.

As stated earlier, a lot has been learned about AIDS in a relatively short time. There has been a lot of excitement, but so far no cure or vaccine has been found; there is not even an effective treatment. Scientists and other professionals are working hard to find ways to halt this dreadful pandemic. Meanwhile, the number of cases is fast increasing; thousands of people are dying; and the infection is spreading to countries and communities where it did not exist before. But there seems to be a lot of hope; and hope is very much displayed at the annual international conferences. Those working hard to halt the pandemic should be given the encouragement and resources to carry on their tasks.

## REFERENCES

Acquired immunodeficiency syndrome (AIDS) among blacks and Hispanics: United States. (1986). *MMWR, 35,* 655-658, 663-666.

Bakeman, R., et al. (1986). AIDS risk-group profiles in whites and members of minority groups. *The New England Journal of Medicine, 315,* 191-192.

Burke, D. S., et al. (1987). HIV infection among civilian application for United States military service: October 1985 to March 1986. *The New England Journal of Medicine, 317,* 131-136.

Clumeck, N., et al. (1983). Acquired immunodeficiency syndrome in black Africans. *Lancet, 1,* 642.

Curran, J. W., et al. (1984). Acquired immunodeficiency syndrome (AIDS) associated with transfusions. *The New England Journal of Medicine, 310,* 69-75.

Curran, J. W., et al. (1988). Epidemiology of HIV infection and AIDS in the United States. *Science, 239,* 610-616.

Fauci, A. S., et al. (1984). Acquired immunodeficiency syndrome: Epidemiologic, clinical, immunologic, and therapeutic considerations. *Annals of Internal Medicine, 100,* 92-106.

Francis, D. P., & Chin, J. (1987). The prevention of acquired immunodeficiency in the United States. *JAMA, 257,* 1357-1365.

Friedland, G. H., & Klein, R. S. (1987). Transmission of the human immunodeficiency virus. *The New England Journal of Medicine, 317,* 1125-1135.

Leads from the *MMWR:* Update—acquired immunodeficiency syndrome—United States. (1987). *JAMA, 257,* 433-437.

Opportunistic infection and Kaposi's sarcoma among Haitians in the United States. (1982). *MMWR, 31,* 353-361.

Peterson, J., & Bakerman, R. (1988). The epidemiology of adult minority AIDS. *Multicultural Inquiry and Research on AIDS, 2,* 1-2.

*Pneumocystis* pneumonia: Los Angeles. (1981). *MMWR, 30,* 250-252.

Quinn, T. C., et al. (1988). Human immunodeficiency virus among patients attending clinics for sexually transmitted diseases. *The New England Journal of Medicine, 318,* 197-202.

Reports on selected racial/ethnic groups. (1988). *MMWR, 37,* 1-3.

Update on Kaposi's sarcoma and opportunistic infections in previously healthy persons: United States. (1982). *MMWR, 31,* 294-301.

# 4

# Transmission of HIV and Pathogenesis of AIDS

As stated in the last chapter, one of the first things established about AIDS was the means of transmission. Even before the causative agent was discovered, it was quite clear that the disease could be contracted in relatively few ways. There has been a lot of discussion about so-called casual transmission, but so far all the evidence points toward four means of transmission: (a) sexual (both homosexual and heterosexual) activity, (b) IV drug use, (c) transfusion of blood/blood products, and (d) from mother to child through the birth process. These four means exist anywhere in the world where there have been AIDS cases, though there is variation in different geographic areas.

The WHO has identified three patterns of transmission worldwide, which have influenced the epidemics of the disease in different geographic areas:

*Pattern 1.* Most cases of AIDS occur in homosexual/bisexual men and IV drug users. Heterosexual transmission is responsible for relatively few cases, although the rate of heterosexual transmission is increasing. Consequently, the majority of AIDS cases are men. The overall national infection rate is probably less than 1% with certain segments of the population having rates in excess of 50%. The United States, most European countries, and some Latin American countries appear to follow this pattern.

*Pattern 2.* Most cases occur in heterosexuals. Transmission through homosexual/bisexual activity and IV drug use is rare. Consequently, male-to-female ratio of AIDS cases approximates 1. The overall national infection rate is probably more than 1% and may exceed 15% in the sexually active young adult populations of some urban areas. Most African countries and several Latin American countries appear to follow this pattern.

*Pattern 3*. HIV has only recently been introduced to these countries. The majority of cases originated outside the country. No homosexual/IV drug use or heterosexual transmission pattern has emerged. The majority of Asian countries, countries in North Africa and most countries in Oceania follow this pattern (WHO Special Programme on AIDS, 1987).

The WHO's patterns of transmission described above seem to reinforce the widely held view that HIV is transmitted through different means and unique individual or group characteristics. When AIDS was first discovered only in homosexual men, it was believed that there was something unique about homosexual activity that promoted transmission and pathogenesis. The same assumption was made about IV drug users. Then it became clear that AIDS occurs in heterosexuals also. Finally, when AIDS in Africa was found in predominantly heterosexual populations, there was speculation about some unique African heterosexual activity that promotes HIV transmission. I maintain that there is one common route of transmission of HIV, whether the means is sexual or otherwise. The route of transmission of HIV is through the blood.

Every time I make an oral presentation on AIDS, I start with this statement: "AIDS has 'nothing' to do with sex, IV drug use, or race." I qualify it by saying that the statement is not entirely true; then I explain the statement in this manner. Transmission of HIV from one person to another is not based on simple sexual intercourse; it is based on access to the bloodstream of the person receiving the virus. By the same token, the mere use of IV drugs has nothing to do with HIV transmission; it is the sharing of needles—indeed, the sharing of blood—that effects transmission. And there is nothing inherent in certain racial groups that promotes transmission. Racial differences in AIDS/HIV-infection prevalence have to do with relative efficiency of access to people's blood by HIV.

## MECHANISM OF HIV TRANSMISSION

Based on basic microbiology and infectious disease principles, three factors must be satisfied before a microorganism is transmitted from one person to another: (a) There has to be a portal of exit, (b) there has to be a medium of survival, and (c) there has to be a portal of entry. For example, a person with a cold sneezes and releases thousands of viruses from the nose (portal of exit) into the surrounding air; the viruses stay alive in the air (medium of survival) for a few seconds; and a susceptible person close by inhales the virus-saturated air through the nose and mouth (portal of entry). The viruses eventually find their way to various body parts and cause the same cold symptoms in the susceptible person. Obviously, the portal of entry is the most important step in the transmission process. In HIV transmission, all evidence indicates that the bloodstream is the portal of entry.

## Sexual Transmission

I maintain that there is no difference in the efficiency of HIV transmission by homosexual and heterosexual activity as long as there is equal access to blood. In the United States and other countries where homosexual transmission far exceeds that of heterosexuals, there is better access to blood in homosexuals. Regarding receptive (penile-vaginal and penile-anal) intercourse, assume that the portal of exit is the same for both homosexuals and heterosexuals. The difference lies in the medium of survival and portal of entry.

The vagina has a very low pH (i.e., it is very acidic). This and other natural secretions make the vaginal environment rather inhospitable, and HIV does not survive very long there. The natural protection in the anus is not that efficient. Next, the vaginal mucosa is lined by a membrane called stratified squamous epithelium. In the presence of normal lubrication, this membrane is rather resistant to lacerations. The anus, on the other hand, is lined by a different membrane, called columnar epithelium. This membrane is friable and breaks more easily. Also, blood vessels are near the surface of the anus, so membrane breakage leads to easy access to blood. Furthermore, the anal opening is very small and quite tight, and insertion of a penis necessarily involves some degree of force, which makes laceration easier. Therefore, both medium of survival and portal of entry are better in anal intercourse, and it has nothing to do with sexual practice; that is, the same risk exists for female or male anal recipients.

Other evidence for efficient portal of entry is the fact that, in strictly penile-vaginal intercourse, transmission is easier from male to female. The act of sexual intercourse, with piston and socket kind of action, makes the vaginal mucosa more likely to tear. Despite the fact that the vaginal mucosa is quite resilient, small tears can occur during intercourse. In addition, the vagina has a wide surface area so that small tears over this large area make for a good portal of entry.

The final evidence lies in the relation between sexually transmitted diseases (STDs) and HIV transmission. Studies have demonstrated high HIV seroprevalence rates in people with STDs. Here, again, the reason is blood. Genital lesions such as chancre (syphilis), chancroid, and genital herpes make for easy access to blood. Also, STDs like gonorrhea and chlamydia produce inflammation that compromises the integrity of vaginal and urethral mucosa and creates access to the bloodstream. Therefore, the existence of STDs creates risk for HIV transmission whether the exposure is to a man or woman.

Portal of entry, such as access to blood, then explains the transmission patterns between homosexuals and heterosexuals and between male and female heterosexuals. But what about the situation in Africa, where heterosexual activity is believed to be the main means of transmission and the male-to-female ratio is about 1? The situation in Africa too complex to be explained by heterosexual activity alone. As will be discussed in the next chapter, the role of STDs, use of inadequately screened donated blood, use of contaminated needles for injection, and certain cultural practices all contribute to the ratio of unity.

What I have implied in the above discussion is that having sex with someone, male or female, with HIV infection will not necessarily lead to the transmission of the virus if there is no access to blood. But this is a big *if*. As discussed above, various conditions or practices can produce access to the bloodstream. And it is sometimes difficult to tell whether you or your partner has a genital tear, genital ulcer, or some other STD. The argument necessarily follows that, the more tears or STDs there are, the more likely transmission is.

This leads to another principle of infectious disease: dose and effect; that is, the larger the dose (of the viruses), the easier the transmission. A large dose could be a large number of viruses deposited at one time or an accumulation of viruses over time. Therefore, if there is an excessive number of viruses, transmission can occur even in the case of very small tears or ulcers. Thus repeated exposure to HIV, as may occur in prostitutes or some homosexuals, is a major risk for transmission. The average homosexual in the United States who has AIDS has had 300 lifetime sex partners. The CDC reported in 1987 a seroprevalence study in a Minnesota social club. The purpose of the club was to exchange sex partners, and members comprised married couples and single individuals. None of 75 men tested was positive, and 2 of 59 women tested were positive for HIV antibodies. The two women had each had repeated sex with more than 25 male members of the club. This illustrates that frequent vaginal intercourse can lead to significant breaks in vaginal mucosa, and exposure to many different sexual partners increases the risk of exposure to HIV.

## Transmission Through Blood and Blood Products

Transfusion of whole blood, blood cell components, plasma, and clotting factors have all been involved in the transmission of HIV. Based on the argument above, transfusion should be and is the easiest way of transmitting HIV. Blood or blood products serve as both the portal of exit and the medium of survival; and this portal of entry, the recipient's bloodstream, is the most direct. Also, dose effect is important here. Transfusion of a pint or more of blood, if infected with HIV, introduces a large number of viruses into the recipient's bloodstream at one time. And transfusion of HIV-infected blood almost always results in HIV infection. This occurs whether the donor blood contains cell-free viruses or cell-associated viruses.

Hemophiliacs basically survive on frequent transfusion of clotting factors. These factors are extracted from many pints of blood and involve many different donors. Therefore, before different ways were used to treat the clotting factors, a lot of transfused factors were infected with HIV. Again, the clotting factors serve as the portal exit and medium of survival for HIV, and the portal of entry for the recipient is direct. Earlier studies showed that 70% to 80% of hemophiliacs were infected with HIV. In recent years, these rates are much lower because of effective treatment of the factors. Heat treatment of the factors kills HIV; and the use of this technique before their transfusion has virtually eliminated HIV-infected factors.

It should be obvious that any blood-to-blood contact could result in transmission. Therefore, sharing of IV drug needles, accidental needle-stick, and injection with unsterile needles can all transmit HIV. The rate of transmission depends upon the dose. There is usually very little blood, and thus few viruses, at the tip of a needle that accidentally sticks someone. Also, a significant amount of time may elapse between the needle's leaving the infected person and the accidental stick. The virus may not survive that long. Furthermore, the accidental needle-stick may not be deep enough for direct bloodstream exposure.

In this regard, studies have shown, after the testing of hundreds of health care workers who accidentally stick themselves, that this route is very inefficient for transmitting HIV. A particular study conducted at the National Institutes of Health found only 3 of more than 500 employees with accidental needle-stick to be positive for HIV antibodies, and they all had had other risks for HIV infection. More important, 50 of the seronegative employees had been stuck with needles known to be contaminated by HIV.

## Transmission Through IV Drug Use

As stated earlier, the risk of transmission of HIV infection through drug use has to do with sharing of blood, not the drug use per se. In other words, if one uses IV drugs and does not share equipment—indeed, does not share blood—there is no risk of contracting HIV. I have visited drug shooting galleries, and it is clear from observation that blood is the route of transmission. Even if equipment were shared without sharing blood, the risk would be much lower.

When drug users meet to indulge themselves, there is a long process of cooking the drug, drawing it into syringes, and injecting the drug. It usually starts with the powdered form of the drug, which is then mixed with water and cooked so it will dissolve as much as possible. Much of the time, it does not dissolve completely so that, when drawn into the syringe, little pellets of the drug stick to the syringe. Keeping in mind that it cost a lot of money to buy the drug, the user wants to get every little bit into his or her body. When the needle is placed into a vein, the user draws blood from the vein into the syringe to pick up the little pellets of drug sticking to walls of the syringes and then pushes the whole syringe back into the vein. The syringe and needle are then passed on to the next person, who does the same thing.

What happens at the drug scene as described above is sharing of blood. When the first user draws his or her own blood into the syringe and pushes it back into his or her vein, some droplets of blood are left inside the syringe and on the tip of the needle. When the next person draws his or her blood into the same syringe, it mixes with the first person's blood before being injected. Obviously, if the preceding blood is infected with HIV, it is transmitted to the succeeding users of the same syringe. Like the situation in blood transfusion, blood serves as portal exit and medium of survival for HIV; the portal of entry is direct. There may not be a large number of viruses injected at any one time, but the frequency with which the sharing goes on causes a very efficient means of HIV transmission.

## Perinatal Transmission

Most AIDS cases and HIV infection in infants and small children occur through maternal transmission during pregnancy or delivery. A pregnant woman infected with HIV may transmit the virus to the fetus through maternal circulation or during labor and delivery by inoculation of maternal blood. Intrauterine infection has been demonstrated by infection in infants delivered by cesarean section and the isolation of HIV from umbilical cord blood. This, of course, is an efficient means of transmission because of the sharing of blood by mother and fetus.

It is important to understand the concept of passive immunity. If a pregnant woman has any type of infection and her body builds antibodies to the infecting agents, those antibodies may be passed on to her fetus. Indeed, infants are protected from most infections by maternal antibodies until their immune systems become mature. Usually, the infant has no effective immune system and is protected by maternal antibodies (passive immunity) until about 6 months after birth. Therefore, when an infant tests positive at birth for antibodies to HIV, he or she should be retested after 6 months. The infant really should be tested every 3 months thereafter for about 15 months. If the initial antibody test were a result of passive immunity, succeeding tests should be negative. If the child tests consistently negative through 15 months of age, it should be considered HIV negative, *provided* he or she shows no signs and symptoms of HIV infection.

## Is There "Casual" Transmission?

One of the major issues about the AIDS epidemic is so-called casual transmission. People have demanded proof that it is not transmitted through handshakes, food or drink, toilet seats, sharing of cooking and eating utensils, and, perhaps the most controversial, insect bites. Although no one can prove that transmission does not occur through these casual means, many studies have clearly demonstrated that it is highly unlikely. Almost every case of AIDS or HIV infection has occurred through some close contact between the infected person and the recipient of the virus.

There have been reports of isolation of HIV from blood, semen, vaginal secretions, saliva, tears, urine, cerebrospinal fluid, and breast milk. Only blood and semen have been demonstrated to involve transmission. The concentration of the viruses in these body fluids is usually too low for effective transmission. Furthermore, my contention is that there has to be direct contact of these with blood for effective transmission and infection. I should mention that there has been one reported case of transmission through breast milk. In that case, the mother became infected with HIV from blood transfusion after delivering the baby. When the baby was later found to be infected also, it was found that the mother had breast-fed the baby for six weeks and HIV was isolated from her breast milk. This led to the conclusion that breast-feeding was the likely route of transmission.

AIDS patients who have spit on people (usually police or prison officers) have been prosecuted for "criminal intent" to transmit "AIDS." Though HIV has been isolated from saliva, no cases of HIV transmission through saliva have been reported. Indeed, there is evidence that saliva may be protective against HIV. Researchers at the National Institute of Dental Research have demonstrated that saliva protected lymphocytes from being infected by HIV. They incubated HIV in saliva with lymphocytes, and the lymphocytes were completely protected from infection. Even when they diluted the saliva at 1:20, it still exhibited about 50% protection. The researchers concluded that there may be "a natural, non-toxic product" in saliva that may have "potential therapeutic benefits" (Fettrer, 1990). The researchers are working on isolating the chemical in saliva that causes the protective effect. According to Dr. Philip Fox, one of the researchers: "Based on what we've seen and the years of experience, there's enough background to say [that saliva] isn't a route of transmission (Fettrer, 1990, p. 109).

I have always tried to avoid the labels *intimate* and *casual* in discussing the transmission of HIV. There is nothing intimate about receiving blood transfusion or clotting factors; neither is there much intimacy in using unsterile syringes and needles. What is important is blood contact by a free virus or virus-infected cells. By the same token, "casual" transmission can occur without intimate contact as is possible from splashes of infected blood.

I had talked about this type of casual transmission for months before the CDC reported three cases of HIV infection in health care workers through this means. My argument was and is that, if there is direct contact with blood by infected blood or other body fluids, transmission can occur. Therefore, a cut on the skin or an ulcer on the skin and other mucous membranes can effect the transmission. It does not have to involve sexual contact or needle-stick.

The CDC reported in July 1987 that three health care workers had tested positive for HIV antibodies and none of the cases involved needle-stick. All three had denied exposure to the virus through any of the recognized means of transmission. One of them had kept a finger on a bleeding artery for about 20 minutes. The other two had blood splashed on their skin or possibly into their mouths or eyes. All three involved patients with documented HIV infection, and all three tested negative but later seroconverted to positive. And all three reportedly had some skin lesions, making blood-to-blood contact rather easy.

If my argument that blood is *the* route of transmission is correct, then it should be expected that the relative efficiency of transmission is higher from blood/blood product transfusion, from use of unsterile syringes and needles, and from mother to infant. It should be relatively less efficient through sexual transmission. This is because, in the former instances, the middle step (medium of survival) in the transmission process is bypassed. Studies have shown that transfusion of infected blood/blood products leads to infection in the recipients 90% of the time; in perinatal transmission, it is 40% to 50%; and in a single sexual contact, it is 0.1%. Obviously, repeated sexual contact, type of sexual activity (rectal versus vaginal), and existence of STDs substantially increase the chance of sexual transmission of the virus. Furthermore, the dose of viruses delivered at one time or the accumulation thereof is of paramount importance.


## PATHOGENESIS OF AIDS

Acquired immunodeficiency syndrome (AIDS) is a new health condition. It results from inability or impaired ability of the immune system to do its job of protecting its victims from various diseases. In other words, the immune system is deficient—hence the name *immunodeficiency*. A *syndrome* is a collection of symptoms or diseases. Therefore, AIDS is really not a disease but a number of different diseases all resulting from a common cause.

There is nothing new about immune deficiency in medical science. Some people are born with various degrees of immune system impairment such that, although they survive rather well, they are unable to fight certain specific infections. Childhood diseases such as Bruton's disease, Di George syndrome, and Chedak-Higashi syndrome all involve immune system impairment. Total lack of immune system function is incompatible with life. Children born with combined immune system (CIDS) disease die early in childhood from simple infections— infections that are otherwise relatively benign.

The important thing about immune deficiency is that it does not kill the victims directly but leaves them "naked" to be attacked by all kinds of infectious agents. Therefore, if a child with CIDS were protected from exposure to infectious agents, he or she might live a full life span. A child named David in Houston was such a patient. He was kept in a plastic bubble soon after birth, and meticulous hygiene was maintained in handling him. He lived to be 12 years old at which time he received a bone marrow transplant. Evidently, the transplant did not produce enough cells for effective immune system, and he died after being taken out of the bubble. AIDS is like CIDS; the difference is that, in the case of AIDS, the person is born with an intact immune system. He or she acquires—hence the name *acquired*— something that destroys the immune system to the point of his or her becoming "naked"; that is, he or she is exposed to and can die from usually benign conditions.

People can acquire immune deficiency but usually not to the degree of devastation as in AIDS. This usually occurs with certain chemotherapeutic medications, corticosteroid, certain types of cancer, and renal disease. Such patients can usually be managed by aggressive antibiotic therapy, and they survive when the implicated drug is withheld. The unique thing about AIDS is that the immune system is destroyed by a virus to the point of rendering the victim helpless to the disease process. Also unique is the fact that the virus seems to have appeared from nowhere. This new disease, acquired immunodeficiency syndrome, has been very well studied during its relatively short history.

Before HIV was discovered, AIDS was defined by the presence, in a previously healthy person less than 60 years old, of

(1) no known cause of immunosuppression such as neoplastic disease, renal failure, or corticosteroid therapy and
(2) a disease predictive of cellular immune dysfunction such as Kaposi's sarcoma, *Pneumocystis carinii* pneumonia, and oral candidiasis.

Since the discovery of HIV, testing positive for antibodies to HIV or recovery of the virus from a person has been added. The question now is this: How does HIV cause immune system impairment leading to the development of those diseases?

Human beings are protected from infectious agents by two major barriers. The skin and mucous membranes provide the first line of defense, and the immune system takes over the fight once the offending agents enter the body. Most organisms cannot penetrate the intact skin; and the various orifices of the body are covered by mucous membranes that provide the same protection as the skin. When the integrity of the skin and mucous membranes is compromised, certain organisms can enter the body. And some other organisms can penetrate intact skin or mucous membranes. Once access to the body has been achieved by the organisms, the various types of ammunition of the immune system are called into play.

Organisms usually travel through lymphatic channels to the bloodstream and then to various tissues in the body. Depending upon the type of organism, it may cause damage to outside cells or invade cells. If the organisms are able to overcome cells in the lymphatic channels, they are attacked by circulating cells called *phagocytes* in the bloodstream. If they are able to reach tissues, tissue phagocytes called *macrophages* then attack the organism. At this level, more ammunition in the immune system is called upon. Special white blood cells called *lymphocytes* come to the aid of the macrophages to effect destruction of the organisms. Whether the body is able to conquer the organisms through this process depends upon the number (dose effect) and virulence (strength) of the invading organisms versus the number and quality (strength) of the various cell types doing the fighting. And, if the body "loses the war," the organisms cause damage to tissues and cells; the person then develops symptoms characteristic of the disease caused by that particular organism.

There are two types of lymphocytes—B lymphocytes and T lymphocytes (or B cells and T cells). They function in a complex manner, but, in general, B cells are involved in the destruction of organisms that cause damage outside cells; T cells attack organisms that invade cells. In general, B cells produce antibodies for the destruction of bacteria; T cells involve the destruction of viruses, parasites, and fungi. The production of antibodies by B cells also requires the assistance of T cells. There are three types of T cells: natural killer cells, T helper cells (T4), and T suppressor cells (T8). T4 plays the most important role in the immune process. As mentioned, it is required by B cells to produce antibodies; it also assists the phagocytic cells, directs destruction of certain organisms, and directs antibody production by the T-cell systems—hence the name *helper*. In effect, the whole immune system is dependent upon T helper cells. HIV specifically attacks these T helper cells.

As stated before, HIV belongs to a group of viruses called *retroviruses*. These are a special type of RNA viruses with the unique ability to reproduce themselves through a DNA intermediate. They utilize an enzyme called *reverse transcriptase*, which produces the DNA intermediate called *provirus*. The provirus is integrated into the cell DNA of a person infected with the retrovirus (the host). The host DNA then effects the production of a new RNA virus (retrovirus). In other words, the retrovirus impregnates the host cell to give birth to another retrovirus. In the process, the host cell dies. HIV is so dangerous because, of the numerous types of cells in the human body, it selectively uses T4 (the most important cell in the immune system) to reproduce itself.

In addition to T4, HIV also is believed to infect macrophages and brain cells. But the main devastation by HIV is the progressive destruction of T4 cells. The average adult has about 1,600 T4 cells per deciliter of blood serum. Once HIV infection occurs in an individual, its progressive destruction of T4 cells is relentless; antibodies are made against HIV but they do not seem to be protective. The rate of destruction of T4 cells depends upon individual characteristics. Therefore, the interval between infection and development of AIDS varies from individual to individual. In general, when the T4-cell level in blood serum drops from the average 1,600 to less than 200 per deciliter, AIDS symptoms develop. The patient develops both common and unusual infections and certain cancers. In addition, some patients develop neurologic disease as a consequence of direct destruction of brain cells by HIV.

The progression from HIV infection to AIDS depends upon how fast the body's immune system is destroyed. The rate of destruction depends upon the number of viruses versus the number and quality of T4 cells in the body. The status of the whole immune system, including T4 cells, is related to the general health of the individual, nutritional status, environmental stress, and the existence of certain other diseases. In addition, lymphocytes, like other cells in the body, undergo constant turnover; that is, old ones die and are replaced by new ones. The liver is the "factory" where raw materials are made for the manufacture of cells and other tissues. Therefore, a healthy liver contributes to the status of the immune system.

What has been discussed in the last chapter implies that a person infected with HIV is likely to progress to AIDS if

(1) his or her general health status is poor;

(2) he or she has poor nutritional status, particularly lack of adequate protein intake;

(3) he or she is under significant environmental stress; or

(4) he or she has coexisting diseases, particularly certain infectious diseases that tend to stimulate the immune system.

A lot of discussion has gone on in regard to the fourth point above, the so-called cofactor issue in the pathogenesis of AIDS. Many studies have demonstrated the existence of such infections as syphilis, cytomegalovirus (CMV), Epstein-Barr virus (EBV), and herpes simplex virus in populations with high rates of HIV infection and AIDS. It is suggested that exposure to these and other infectious agents causes the immune system to be chronically activated and thereby makes it more susceptible to HIV infection and lymphocyte destruction. This is based on laboratory evidence that lymphocytes that are activated replicate viruses more efficiently.

A study reported in the *Journal of the American Medical Association* (Quinn et al., 1987) found a high rate of these infections in many AIDS patients. They found high antibody levels for CMV, EBV, hepatitis A and B, herpes simplex virus, syphilis, and toxoplasmosis in 38 African and 60 U.S. patients with AIDS. There was no significant difference in the prevalence of antibodies to these infectious agents between the two groups. They also tested 100 African and 100 U.S. heterosexual and 100 U.S. homosexuals without AIDS or antibodies to these agents. The results showed no significant difference between the AIDS patients and the 100 African heterosexuals and 100 U.S. homosexuals. However, the prevalence of antibodies to these agents was significantly lower in the 100 U.S. heterosexuals without AIDS than in the other groups.

This study illustrates the likely relationship between frequent or chronic exposure to certain infectious agents and the pathogenesis of AIDS.

Two groups, African heterosexuals (at least Africans in Central Africa, where the study was done) and U.S. homosexuals, with a high rate of AIDS were found to have a high rate of antibodies to many infectious agents. On the other hand, the prevalence of AIDS is relatively low among U.S. heterosexuals; the prevalence of antibodies to those infectious agents is also relatively low. The study lends much credence to the cofactor theory. However, the dose effect is very important.

I have discussed the dose effect in my oral presentations using what I call the "dam theory." A dam is erected to hold water at bay. Rain could cause flooding on the other side of the dam based on the height of the dam and intensity of the rain.

(1) If it rains in moderate amounts and the dam is relatively tall, there will be flooding.
(2) If it rains in moderate amounts and the dam is relatively short, there will be flooding.
(3) If it rains in very large amounts (either heavily one time or moderately over several days) and the dam is relatively tall, flooding can occur.
(4) If it rains in very large amounts and the dam is relatively short, there will be flooding.

The dam theory could help sort out why some people take a relatively long time to develop AIDS after HIV infection and others get AIDS rather quickly. Those with relatively tall dams (strong immune systems) and moderate rain (moderate number of viruses) take a long time to develop AIDS or may never get AIDS. On the other hand, those with relatively short dams (weaker immune systems) but large amounts of rain (larger number of viruses) get AIDS relatively quickly.

The dam theory applies irrespective of group or individual behavior as already discussed in this chapter. Whether homosexual or heterosexual, whether through blood transfusion or IV drug use, AIDS symptoms are likely to occur if "the amount of rain is large enough to cause flooding."

## CLINICAL MANIFESTATIONS OF AIDS

Once a person is infected with HIV, there is a progression from the initial infection to the development of AIDS (see Figure 4.1). The initial

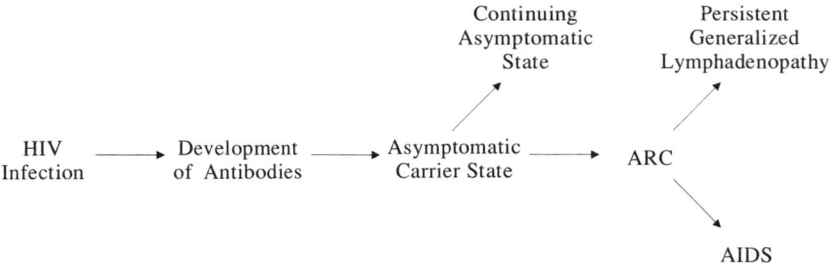

**Figure 4.1**. Natural History of HIV Infection

infection may or may not produce flulike symptoms—headache, body aches, fatigue, fever. This illness is very nonspecific because most viruses, including those that cause the common cold, produce the same symptoms; and the illness may last only a few days with full recovery. As more lymphocytes are destroyed, the patient may develop AIDS-related complex (ARC) and, finally, AIDS. It should be borne in mind that some people do not have the initial flulike illness or develop ARC; they are diagnosed with AIDS at the first presentation for medical care. ARC is characterized by any two of the following:

(1) unexplained lymphadenopathy (involving lymph nodes on various parts of the body),
(2) fever of unknown origin for at least three weeks,
(3) unexpected diarrhea for at least two months leading to a weight loss of at least 10 kg (about 22 pounds),
(4) unexplained fatigue for at least three weeks, and
(5) oral candidiasis (yeast infection of the mouth and throat).

There are three main clinical characteristics of AIDS resulting from the destruction of lymphocytes and other cells:

(1) unusual cancers:
    (a) Kaposi's sarcoma
    (b) certain lymphomas
(2) constitutional symptoms:
    (a) fever, decreased (or lack of) appetite, fatigue, weight loss

(b) opportunistic infections

(3) AIDS dementia

The clinical manifestations of AIDS outlined above are a reflection of an impaired immune system. Characteristically, some of these symptoms are displayed by some old people because there seems to be immune system impairment with the normal aging process. The difference is that these illnesses are usually inconsequential because immune system impairment with normal aging does not occur to the same degree observed with AIDS. For example, Kaposi's sarcoma is a relatively benign cancer commonly found in some African and Mediterranean populations. It usually affects people more than 60 years old, and it normally does not cause death. With AIDS, however, the patients are much younger and often die from the cancer. In addition, dementia is often an illness of old people. However, because of destruction of brain cells by HIV, young people with AIDS may develop dementia. Indeed, dementia may be the first clinical presentation after HIV infection.

The other major clinical manifestation of AIDS is opportunistic infections. As stated earlier, these infections usually cause self-limiting illnesses; however, they can cause major problems in the presence of immune system impairment. Because AIDS results from total immune system impairment, AIDS patients develop opportunistic infections with organisms from all major microbial groups:

(1) Protozoa: *Pneumocystis carinii,* toxoplasma, cryptosporidium, giardia, amoeba

(2) Fungi: candida, cryptococcus, coccidioidomycosis

(3) Viruses: cytomegalovirus (CMV), Epstein-Barr virus (EBV), herpes simplex, herpes zoster

(4) Bacteria: *Mycobacterium tuberculosis, Mycobacterium avium intracellulare,* salmonella

Opportunistic infections cause most of the deaths in AIDS patients, and *Pneumocystis carinii* pneumonia is the most common type of opportunistic infection causing death. However, all the organisms listed above (and others) usually contribute to the debilitation of AIDS patients. A point of interest is the fact that, although some of these organisms—CMV, EBV, herpes simplex, toxoplasma—cause disease in AIDS patients, it is suggested that individuals who had been exposed to these organisms before HIV infection tend to progress more

**Table 4.1**   Revised Definition of AIDS (CDC, 1987)

---

*If laboratory tests for HIV were not performed or gave inconclusive results and the patient had no other cause of immunodeficiency, then any disease listed below indicates AIDS if it was diagnosed by a definitive method.*

---

1. Candidiasis of the esophagus, trachea, bronchi, or lungs
2. Cryptococcosis, extrapulmonary
3. Cryptosporidiosis with diarrhea persisting over 1 month
4. Cytomegalovirus disease of an organ other than liver, spleen, or lymph nodes in a patient over 1 month of age
5. Herpes simplex virus infection causing a mucocutaneous ulcer that persists longer than 1 month; or bronchitis, pneumonitis, or esophagitis for any duration affecting a patient over 1 month of age
6. Kaposi's sarcoma affecting a patient under 60 years of age
7. Lymphoma of the brain (primary) affecting a patient under 60 years of age
8. Lymphoid interstitial pneumonia and/or pulmonary lymphoid hyperplasia affecting a child under 13 years of age
9. *Mycobacterium avium* complex or *M. Kansasii* disease at sites other than or in addition to lungs, skin, or cervical or hilar lymph nodes
10. *Pneumocystis carinii* pneumonia
11. Progressive multifocal leukoencephalopathy
12. Toxoplasmosis of the brain affecting a patient over 1 month of age

---

SOURCE: U.S. Centers for Disease Control (1987).

quickly to AIDS. In other words, these organisms are cofactors of HIV infection in the pathogenesis of AIDS and also cause opportunistic infections in AIDS symptomatology.

A word about tuberculosis (TB). Several types of mycobacteria cause respiratory and other illnesses but *Mycobacterium tuberculosis* is the best known and the most pathogenic. In any case, all the mycobacteria tend to be opportunistic; they are more dangerous in individuals with some degree of immune system impairment. Therefore, at least in developed nations, TB is most common in children less than 5 years old (whose immune system is not fully developed yet) and older people over 60 years (who have immune system impairment through the aging process). The TB organisms may stay in the body without causing disease, kept in check by the immune system; then they may cause disease when the immune system becomes impaired. Therefore, TB in older people usually reflects reactivation of dormant TB organisms instead of new infection.

**Table 4.2**   Revised Definition of AIDS (CDC, 1987)

*Regardless of the presence of other causes of immunodeficiency, in the presence of laboratory evidence for HIV infection, disease listed in Table 4.1 or below indicates a diagnosis of AIDS.*

Indicator diseases diagnosed definitively
 1. bacterial infections, multiple or recurrent (any combination of at least two within a 2-year period) of following types affecting a child under 13 years of age: septicemia, pneumonia, meningitis, bone or joint infection, or abscess of an internal organ or mucosal abscesses caused by *Haemophilus, Streptococcus* (including pneumococcus), or other pyogenic bacteria;
 2. coccidioidomycosis, disseminated (at a site other than or in addition to lungs or cervical or hilar lymph nodes);
 3. HIV encephalopathy (also called "HIV dementia," "AIDS dementia" or "subacute encephalitis due to HIV");
 4. histoplasmosis at sites other than or in addition to lungs or cervical or hilar lymph nodes;
 5. isosporiasis with diarrhea persisting over 1 month;
 6. Kaposi's sarcoma at any age;
 7. lymphoma of the brain (primary) at any age;
 8. other non-Hodgkin's lymphoma of B-cell or unknown immunological phenotype;
 9. any mycobacterial disease caused by mycobacteria other than *M. tuberculosis* at sites other than or in addition to lungs, skin, or cervical or hilar lymph nodes;
10. disease caused by *M. tuberculosis* at sites outside the lungs, regardless of whether there is concurrent pulmonary involvement;
11. *Salmonella* (nontyphoid) septicemia, recurrent; and
12. HIV wasting syndrome (emaciation, "slim disease").

SOURCE: U.S. Centers for Disease Control (1987).

The incidence of TB in the United States had been decreasing about 5% yearly since the 1950s until it leveled off in 1985. In 1986, the incidence actually increased by about 2% and has been increasing steadily since. The new cases are not occurring in children under 5 years but in people in their twenties, thirties, and forties. This trend indicated that there was reactivation of dormant TB instead of new infection. Later studies showed that most of the new TB cases were in AIDS patients and individuals with HIV infection. Significantly, TB in AIDS patients tends to occur more in other body organs than in the lung. In addition, less pathogenic mycobacteria like *Mycobacterium avium intracellulare* tend to produce serious illness in AIDS patients. TB is a major opportunistic infection in AIDS patients in Africa. The WHO announced in October 1990 that the incidence of TB is increasing worldwide because of HIV infection; and the WHO was having difficulty raising adequate funds to control it.

The clinical definition of AIDS summarized earlier in this chapter and the symptomatology outlined above are what had been used to diagnose AIDS earlier in the history of the epidemic. Since August 1987, a revised clinical definition for surveillance, developed by the CDC, has been in use. (See Table 4.1 and Table 4.2.) The revised version was developed in response to the need to expand the clinical criteria for diagnosing AIDS. After the discovery of HIV, and when more knowledge became available on the pathogenesis of AIDS, it became clear that other disease processes occur with AIDS in addition to opportunistic infections and certain cancers. The purpose of the expanded definition is to assure more accurate diagnosis and more accurate reporting of the disease. It is estimated that the use of the old definition would miss 10% to 15% of AIDS cases.

## REFERENCES

Biggar, R. J. (1987). AIDS and HIV infection: Estimates of the magnitude of the problem worldwide in 1985/1986. *Clinical Immunology and Immunopathology, 45,* 297-309.

Bolling, R., & Bruce, V. (1987). AIDS and heterosexual anal intercourse. *JAMA, 258,* 474.

Centers for Disease Control. (1987). Revision of the surveillance case definition for acquired immunodeficiency syndrome. *MMWR, 36,* S1-S15.

Fauci, A. S., et al. (1984). Acquired immunodeficiency syndrome: Epidemiologic, clinical, immunologic, and therapeutic considerations. *Annals of Internal Medicine, 100,* 92-106.

Feorino, P. M., Jaffe, H. W., et al. (1985). Transfusion-associated acquired immunodeficiency syndrome: Evidence for persistent infection in blood donors. *The New England Journal of Medicine, 312,* 1293-1296.

Fettrer, A. C. (1990, October 4). Saliva may inhibit HIV. *Medical Tribune,* 109.

Fischl, M. A., Dickinson, G. M., et al. (1987). Evaluation of heterosexual partners, children, and household contacts of adults with AIDS. *JAMA, 257,* 640-644.

Francis, D. P., & Chin, J. (1987). The prevention of AIDS in the U.S.: An objective strategy for medicine, public health, business, and the community. *JAMA, 257,* 1357-1366.

Francis, D. P., Jaffee, H. W., et al. (1985). The natural history of infection with the lymphadenopathy-associated virus/human T-lymphotropic virus type-III. *Annals of Internal Medicine, 103,* 719-722.

Friedland, G. H., Saltzmann, B. R., et al. (1986). Lack of transmission of HTLV-III/ALV infection to household contacts of patients with AIDS or AIDS-related complex with oral candidiasis. *The New England Journal of Medicine, 314,* 344-349.

Fujikawa, L. S., Salahuddin, S. Z., et al. (1985). Isolation of human T-lymphotrophic virus type III from tears of a patient with acquired immunodeficiency syndrome. *Lancet, 2,* 529-530.

Groopman, J. E., Salahuddin, S. Z., et al. (1984). HTLV-III in saliva of people with AIDS-related complex and healthy homosexuals at risk for AIDS. *Science, 226,* 447-449.

Ho, D. D., Byington, R. E., et al. (1985). Infrequency of isolation of HTLV-III virus from saliva in AIDS. *The New England Journal of Medicine, 313,* 1606.

Mann, J. M., Quinn, T. C., et al. (1986). Prevalence of HTLV-III/LAV in household contacts of patients with confirmed AIDS and controls in Kinshasa, Zaire. *JAMA, 256,* 721-724.

Marlink, R. G., & Essex, M. (1987). Africa and the biology of human immunodeficiency virus. *JAMA, 257,* 2632-2633.

Oksenhendler, E., Harzil, M., et al. (1986). HIV infection with seroconversion after a superficial needlestick injury to the finger. *The New England Journal of Medicine, 315,* 582.

Peterman, T., & Curran, J. W. (1986). Sexual transmission of human immunodeficiency virus. *JAMA, 256,* 2222-2226.

Piot, P., & Colebunders, R. (1987). Clinical manifestation and the natural history of HIV infection in adults. *Western Journal of Medicine, 147,* 709-712.

Piot, P., Plummer, F. A., et al. (1987). Retrospective seroepidemiology of AIDS virus infection in Nairobi populations. *The New England Journal of Medicine, 115,* 1108-1112.

Quinn, T. C., Piot, P., et al. (1987). Serologic and immunologic studies in patients with AIDS in North America and Africa: The potential role of infectious agents as co-factors in human immunodeficiency virus infection. *JAMA, 257,* 2617-2621.

Torrey, B. B., Way, P. D., & Rowe, P. M. (1988). Epidemiology of HIV and AIDS in Africa: Emerging issues and social implications. In N. Miller & R. C. Rockwell (Eds.), *AIDS in Africa: The social and policy impact.* Lewiston/Queenston: Edwin Mellen.

Weiss, S. H., Saxinger, W. C., et al. (1985). HTLV-III infection among health care workers: Association with needle-stick injuries. *JAMA, 254,* 2089-2093.

Winkelstein, W., Lyman, D. M., et al. (1987). Sexual practices and risk of infection by human immunodeficiency virus: The San Francisco Men's Study Group. *JAMA, 257,* 321-325.

# 5

---

# AIDS in Africa

Since the time that AIDS cases began to be reported from African countries, there has been controversy and speculation about AIDS in Africa. Two issues of contention are the belief that AIDS in Africa is different than AIDS in other countries and that AIDS (or the virus that causes AIDS) originated in Africa. There has been a lot of discussion on these two issues, particularly the first one.

In March 1987, a group of AIDS experts under the auspices of UNICEF met at the Tufts University European Center in Talloires, France, to discuss AIDS and development. A consensus statement was issued at the end of the meeting, and one of the items was titled "Dangerous Misconceptions," under which this statement appeared:

> There is a widespread myth that AIDS in Africa, and the way it is transmitted, is somehow different from AIDS in developed countries, and therefore causes some special planetary danger. African AIDS is transmitted in exactly the same ways as AIDS in other societies. It does not jump out of trees at visiting tourists or businessmen. We are talking about sex and blood transmission.

The main reason there might be a misconception about AIDS in Africa is the so-called heterosexual transmission there. It has to do with the fact that there is about a 1:1 male-female ratio among African AIDS patients, while the ratio is about 13:1 among U.S. and European patients. The 1:1 ratio in Africa is believed to be due to heterosexual transmission, and the male preponderance in the United States and Europe is believed to be due to homosexual transmission.

As will be discussed later in this chapter, the transmission process in Africa may not only be explained on a sexual basis.

Another point of contention about AIDS being different in Africa is the idea that it is killing millions of people there. There is even speculation that the whole African continent is being lost to AIDS and that nothing much can be done about it. This was said at the UNICEF conference cited above:

> The idea that somehow Africa might already be lost to AIDS . . . is a preposterous idea. Even in African countries where the infection is already real and widespread, it still affects only small numbers relative to the whole population. The idea that a whole generation in some African countries should be written off is acceptable neither in human nor in developmental terms.

In an article in *Lancet,* Dr. Konotey-Ahulu (1987b) of Cromwell Hospital in London discusses his discontent with the idea that AIDS is destroying the whole continent of Africa. He traveled through 16 sub-Saharan African countries to assess the AIDS situation. His report illuminates the profound exaggeration that accompanies many reports on AIDS in Africa. He takes particular issue with labeling the whole continent; there are 51 distinct countries in Africa, and only 5 or 6 have major problems with AIDS. Why are the remaining countries so labeled? He expresses frustration at news reports of rampant deaths from AIDS in Africa: "If tens of thousands are dying from AIDS (and Africans do not cremate their dead) where are the graves?" (Konotey-Ahulu, 1987b, p. 207).

As was evident in the preceding chapter, I completely agree with the pronouncements by the UNICEF group and Dr. Konotey-Ahulu. Indeed, I have been "preaching" on this topic for years. In most of my oral presentations, I take time to discuss AIDS in Africa. I draw the map of Africa and circle the area in East and Central Africa in which most of reported cases in Africa have occurred. I then discuss the prevalence of AIDS in relation to other killer diseases in Africa. Even if one assumes that AIDS is grossly underreported—say only 10% of cases are reported—the death rate from AIDS is still relatively small. For example, malaria kills more than a million people yearly; diarrheal and respiratory illnesses kill even more. Even vaccine-preventable diseases such as measles and tuberculosis kill millions each year. My contention is that AIDS is not killing millions of

Africans *now,* but it has the potential to do just that if the world permits. It is indeed preposterous to write off any African country.

## EPIDEMIOLOGY OF AIDS AND HIV INFECTION IN AFRICA

As of August 31, 1990, 70,724 cases of AIDS have been reported to the WHO from 45 African countries. These represent the cumulative cases since the disease was first recognized on the continent. Of the 45 countries, 24 have reported more than 100 cases, and 9 of those countries have reported more than 1,000 cases. In other terms, only 11 countries have reported more than 10 cases per 100,000 population. Of the nine countries with more than 1,000 total cases, only Ghana and the Côte d'Ivoire are in West Africa; the rest are in Central and contiguous East African countries. In addition, all the countries with more than 10 cases per 100,000 population are located in the latter area of the continent except the Côte d'Ivoire.

The first cases of AIDS were reported in Africa in 1982. It appears that the presence of the disease in Africa parallels that in the United States, suggesting that the virus was introduced to the Americas and Africa at about the same time. However, some studies have suggested that HIV might have been in Africa much earlier. Serologic tests have detected antibody response to blood collected from Zaire in 1959; similar findings have been reported from West and East Africa in the 1960s and early 1970s. These and other earlier studies on HIV-antibody detection in Africa have been questioned because of tests employed and methods used to interpret the results. There appears to be cross-reactivity of the HIV antigen with the antigens of some tropical infectious agents such as the *Plasmodium* (the organism that causes malaria).

In every African country from which AIDS cases have been reported, the geographic distribution has paralleled that in other parts of the world—that is, most cases are in urban areas. However, the two leading risk behaviors for AIDS—homosexual activity and IV drug use—in the Americas and Europe are rare (if not absent) in most African countries. It appears that heterosexual activity is the main means of transmission based on the approximately 1:1 ratio of male-female cases. Studies from several countries indicate that the distribution of AIDS cases based on sex and age group follows that of other sexually transmitted diseases. The contribution of blood transfusion and medical injections is a significant one.

The distribution of HIV infection in African countries closely parallels that of AIDS. Studies from different countries have shown much higher prevalence rates in urban than rural areas. Others with high prevalence rates are prostitutes, patients attending STD clinics, and hospitalized patients. The age group with the highest prevalence of HIV-antibody positivity is the same as that for AIDS. The prevalence of HIV-antibody positivity in infants and very small children in some countries indicates that perinatal transmission is a significant contributor. The prevalence in school-age children is much lower as it is for AIDS cases. Finally, socioeconomic status appears to play a role in the distribution of HIV.

As stated before, most cases of AIDS (and HIV infection) in Africa have occurred in Central and East Africa. West Africa has fewer but significant numbers, and reported cases from North Africa are even fewer. Though the HIV-1 infection rate appears to be low in West Africa, countries in that part of the continent have the highest prevalence of HIV-2. The transmission and pathogenesis of HIV-2 are not as well studied, so the degree of AIDS caused by HIV-2 is not known. However, early indications are that HIV-2 may not be as devastating as HIV-1.

## TRANSMISSION OF HIV-1 IN AFRICA

As discussed in the last chapter, there are four recognized means of transmission of HIV: sexual activity, IV drug use, transfusion of blood/blood products, and perinatally. The same means exist in Africa except for IV drug use. Also, although homosexual activity predominates in the Americas and Europe, heterosexual activity appears to be the sexual means of transmission in Africa. Furthermore, in the absence of IV drug use (and needle sharing), medical injections— what I call "institutional needle sharing"—is a significant contributor to the transmission process.

### Heterosexual Transmission

It is believed that heterosexual activity is the main means of HIV transmission in Africa because of the 1:1 male-female ratio. In addition, both AIDS cases and HIV-infection rates are highest in the most sexually active age groups. Studies from different countries have shown the risk factors accompanying heterosexual activity—increased number of sexual partners, being a prostitute, frequent sexual encounters with prostitutes, and sexual encounters with infected individuals. Significant association with STDs such as gonorrhea, syphilis, and genital ulcers has been demonstrated.

No studies have clearly demonstrated that the 1:1 male-female ratio is due to heterosexual activity. Medical injections and transfusion of blood/blood products may make a significant contribution to such a ratio. Medical injections are so widespread a practice in most African countries that it is a major risk where sterilization of injection equipment is inadequate. And this risk exists for other diseases such as malaria and hepatitis B.

## Medical Injections

There is a widespread belief in many African countries that injected medication is more effective than oral medication. Patients (or parents of pediatric patients) tend to be disappointed when a clinic issues oral medication instead of an injection. Some people even request injections if they are not offered. Preference for injections appears to be present in Latin America also. A friend told me that, in rural Guatemala, not only does an injection have to be given but it should also hurt to be effective. In my work in various STD clinics in Texas, I have had several Mexican natives ask me for a shot of penicillin instead of the oral medication. The use of medical injections in many African countries is not limited to clinics and hospitals. Private individuals, particularly in rural areas, may keep some medication and injection equipment in their homes to give injections to town folk.

In some cases, people giving injections are inadequately trained in aseptic technique; sometimes there are no facilities for adequate sterilization of needles and other injection equipment. Due to lack of financial and other resources, reuse of disposable needles and syringes occurs even in some well-run clinics and hospitals. I visited a rather large clinic in a big city in Africa in December 1987. In a conversation with one of the clinic doctors, she remarked that the doctors in the country were fully aware of the potential danger of reusing disposable needles; "but we cannot, we simply cannot afford to throw needles and syringes away," she added. Because of severe shortages of such equipment in the country, she said, the clinic kept about 100 new syringes and needles on hand; if anyone specifically requested new equipment, it was used. Otherwise, they did the best they could to sterilize disposable needles and syringes for reuse.

I visited another clinic in a different city in the same country in 1982, and what I observed was even more dangerous. This clinic had a long line of people waiting for injected vaccinations. Evidently to save time, the nurse drew enough of the vaccine for several people into a large syringe. He had a piece of cotton in his left hand and the syringe in his right. He would inject so many cc's into one person's shoulder, wipe the spot before and after the shot with the piece of cotton, and immediately do the same to the next person in line until the vaccine in the syringe was finished, which was after four or five individuals. He would use the same needle and syringe to draw the vaccine and start the process again. And the piece of cotton was visibly dirty after a while. Evidently cotton is also a precious commodity in that clinic.

## Blood Transfusions

Although blood and blood product transfusion in the United States and Europe is relatively safe, it is still quite dangerous in terms of HIV transmission in Africa. Many countries lack appropriate resources for effective screening of blood before transfusion. In addition, many endemic illnesses lead to anemia and the need for blood transfusion.

Malnutrition is a significant contributing factor to anemia in some parts of the continent. Endemic diseases such as malaria, tuberculosis, and sickle-cell anemia lead to anemia that may require transfusion. Blood transfusion is often required during delivery of babies. Many poor pregnant women do not have enough nutrient intake to increase their blood volume during pregnancy; some lose a lot of the little blood they have during delivery and require transfusion.

It is obvious that, in the areas of Africa where malaria and tuberculosis are prevalent, the need for blood transfusion is also high. However, screening of donors and the donated blood is inadequate in many of those countries. Processing and storage facilities may be in short supply. Above all, young adults are the most likely to donate blood, and it is they who have the highest prevalence of HIV infection.

**Perinatal Transmission**

As discussed above, the prevalence of AIDS and HIV infection may be rather high in young adults in certain African countries. Women in this age group are the most fertile and are a major source of pediatric AIDS/HIV infection. Maternal transmission of HIV is no different in Africa than it is in the United States and other countries. Studies from different African countries demonstrate a strong association between maternal HIV infection and infant seropositivity. Antibodies to HIV (or the virus itself) may be passed from a mother to the fetus during pregnancy or during delivery through passive transfer of blood. Also, various studies have shown high HIV-antibody rates in pregnant women in certain countries. The seropositive rates in infants born to such women are likely to be high. However, as discussed in the last chapter, a portion of seropositive infants will only possess passively transferred maternal antibodies instead of the virus itself.

## CLINICAL MANIFESTATIONS

The clinical manifestations of AIDS described in the last chapter apply to AIDS patients in African countries. African AIDS patients have Kaposi's sarcoma and other lymphoma and opportunistic infections, as is the case for AIDS patients elsewhere. However, studies indicate that, in Central Africa, dermatological and gastrointestinal problems are more common than the generalized lymphadenopathy and pulmonary problems prevalent in the United States. These manifestations have been observed in Africans living in their native countries and those diagnosed in Europe.

Diagnostic studies in Europe and Africa demonstrate a relation between endemic diseases and the opportunistic infections African AIDS patients tend to possess. The most common infections are oral candidiasis, cryptococcal meningitis, cryptosporidiosis, and herpes simplex virus infection. Other infections include histoplasmosis, salmonellosis, strongyloidiasis, and mycobacterial infections. In contrast, AIDS patients who contracted the disease in the United States and Europe have *Pneumocystis carinii* pneumonia as the predominant opportunistic infection, manifested by nearly 63% of AIDS patients there.

Studies in several Central African countries indicate a relationship between endemic conditions and AIDS symptoms in children. The most common associations are malnutrition and anemia. Malnourished and anemic children tend to have pneumonias, diarrhea, oral candidiasis, lymphadenopathy, and dermatitis more frequently.

## THE ORIGIN OF HIV AND AIDS

Over the years, I have been asked both formally and informally where AIDS originated. I am asked this question to confirm the widely accepted belief that it originated in Africa. I have been asked the question by Africans and Americans. Africans tend to ask angrily whether it is true and ask why the rest of the world wants to blame Africa for everything bad. I usually respond to the Africans by saying it doesn't matter whether it originated in Africa, the issue is where it did originate. To both Africans and Americans, I respond that nobody knows where AIDS originated. I then offer a discussion reflecting my personal belief that it did not originate in Africa. I have been talking about my personal belief for years based on "gut feeling" evidence; recent data demonstrate that I and those who believe the same way are probably right, which will be discussed below.

The belief that AIDS originated in Africa has to do with the discovery in the early 1980s of retroviruses in monkeys from Africa. The early discoveries involved some similarities between monkey retroviruses and human retroviruses. The human retroviruses were isolated from patients with leukemia. When AIDS was recognized as being caused by a retrovirus, questions arose regarding its origin. It was speculated that a similar relationship may exist between monkey retroviruses and HIV—that is, that a monkey retrovirus got into humans somehow and underwent mutation to become HIV.

Initial findings on the relationship between monkey and human retroviruses showed a connection with HTLV-1. This retrovirus isolated from patients with leukemia was found to share certain genes with a retrovirus isolated in the African green monkey. The monkey virus was renamed simian T-lymphotropic virus type I (STLV-1). Antibodies to STLV-1 were detected in the African green monkey in several Central and East African countries in the late 1960s and 1970s. This same virus (STLV-1) was isolated in Asian macaque monkeys, but the one from the African green monkey shared more nucleotide sequences with HTLV-1. Therefore, it was speculated later that HTLV-III (HIV-1) is more likely to have evolved from the African green monkey.

In 1985, another retrovirus was isolated from African green monkeys in the laboratory of Dr. Myron Essex at Harvard University. They named this virus STLV-III because of antigenic similarity between it and HTLV-III. Subsequent studies indicated that the two viruses share about 55% of nucleotide sequences. Also, STLV-III attaches at the CD4 site of lymphocytes as does HTLV-III. The speculation then became that HTLV-III is more likely to have evolved from STLV-III.

Antibodies to STLV-III were detected in many African green monkeys but in none of many chimpanzees and baboons. The infected green monkeys were healthy, implying that STLV-III did not cause disease in the monkeys but is an efficient means of transmission. This discovery lent more credence to the speculation that the monkey virus somehow entered the human body, where the nonpathogenic virus underwent mutation to become the pathogenic HTLV-III. As further evidence for the monkey-human transfer of retroviruses, the African green monkey is known to be more likely than other primates to be in close contact and interact with humans. Also, human blood serum containing antibodies to HIV demonstrated cross-reactivity with that of STLV-III, and the cross-reactions appeared most commonly in blood from Africans.

So the story goes like this: There is close similarity between STLV-III (SIV) and HTLV-III (HIV); SIV is isolated in African green monkeys, and the green monkeys have close contacts with humans in Central and East Africa; the cross-reaction between SIV and HIV is more common to Africans. Therefore, SIV got into humans in Central and East Africa. It underwent mutation to become HIV. Then HIV was imported to the United States and Europe.

But how did SIV get into humans in Africa? How did it get to the United States and Europe? Why was AIDS first recognized in homosexuals when homosexual activity is supposed to be absent in the African populations where HIV is supposed to have originated?

The speculation is that the green monkeys bit humans and transmitted SIV. Alternatively, humans ate green monkeys with SIV infection and thus contracted the virus. SIV underwent mutation to become HIV and somehow maintained a silent infectious state. During the immediate postindependence years (the early 1960s), many of the countries in Central and East Africa required expert knowledge; the experts who came included Haitians. The Haitian experts (mostly men) had sex with African women who were infected with HIV. They returned to Haiti and spread the virus in heterosexual and bisexual populations. Homosexuals from San Francisco went to Haiti on vacation, had sex with infected bisexuals, and contracted the virus. They brought it to San Francisco. Meanwhile, some of the European experts also had sex with infected African women and similarly introduced the virus to the homosexual population in Europe. The virus spread from homosexual IV drug users to heterosexual IV drug users, and then it finally spread to the rest of the population.

The story as I have narrated above has been the "official" scenario of the origins of AIDS/HIV infection. I have heard officials from the CDC give this scenario. I have heard officials of state public health departments give the same scenario. And I have heard infectious disease specialists, recognized in their communities as AIDS experts, give the scenario. The story is told so matter-of-factly that there seems to be no doubt about it. But the story of where HIV originated and how it spread is just that—a *story*. Yet, based on this scenario, it is almost universally accepted that AIDS and the virus that causes it originated in Africans. Both popular and scientific publications espouse this view.

I have been telling my own story about the origins of HIV. I have maintained a belief that HIV is not a new virus; that is, it did not result from the mutation of a monkey virus. It has been present all the time. It had not caused devastating disease and an epidemic because there had not existed the right conditions for viral propagation and transmission.

As stated in the last chapter, the right portal of entry has to exist for the transmission of an organism and establishment of infection. And blood is the portal of entry for HIV. In the 1960s and 1970s, the so-called sexual revolution emerged in the United States and Europe. Casual sexual encounters became the norm, and having several sexual partners was accepted behavior. Significantly, homosexual activity became an open issue; no more did homosexuals have to "hide in the closet." Gay bars and bathhouses became places to pick up sex partners or engage in sexual activity with multiple partners. When I worked in a health department in a large metropolitan area in Florida in 1974, we used to go to a place where homosexuals met to have orgies, every Thursday, to draw blood for serologic tests. In those days, we were concerned about the spread of syphilis.

Concurrent with the sexual revolution was the drug use scene. Many of the same people who indulged in IV drug use also had multiple sexual partners. The so-called drug culture involved sharing of needles and bodies. So the sexual revolution and drug culture combined to create the right environment for HIV to manifest itself as a dangerous virus. Both multiple (and frequent) sexual activity and needle sharing created the ideal portal of entry for the spread of HIV infection and AIDS. Both sexual and needle sharing promoted infection by other agents, many of which effected efficient pathogenesis of HIV and the development of AIDS. The virus was subsequently introduced into Africa.

Why has AIDS spread so quickly in some African countries? My response is that the right conditions existed before the virus was introduced. The presence of STDs, particularly genital ulcers; the frequent use of blood transfusion to treat anemias, particularly those caused by the malaria parasites; and the frequent use of medical injections were "ready made" for fast spread of the virus. In addition, the poor health status of many of the people infected with the virus permitted a rather fast progression to AIDS.

As stated earlier, the view I have espoused on the origin of HIV is not based on hard data. So I was extremely pleased to listen to Dr. Robert Gallo express a similar view during the Fourth International Conference on AIDS in Stockholm, Sweden. Gallo, of the National Cancer Institute and codiscoverer of HIV, presented data to dispute the fact that HIV resulted from the simian equivalent of the African green monkey. He said another simian virus isolated from the Asian velvet monkey was more closely related to HIV than the one from the African green monkey. The Asian monkey virus shares more nucleic acid sequences with HIV; in addition, the Asian SIV, like HIV, has always existed, perhaps confined to a small population of people in whom it had caused low-grade morbidity and mortality. It subsequently spread to other populations and became an epidemic.

In an article published in the *Journal of the National Medical Association,* Katner and Pankey (1987) provide further evidence that HIV did not evolve from the African green monkey. They discount the African origin by pointing out the dissimilarity between HIV and the African SIV. However, there is a much closer similarity between the *visna-maedi* agent and HIV. This agent has been known to infect northern European sheep, and there has been documented sexual contact between male humans and sheep. Furthermore, they describe 28 cases of an aggressive form of Kaposi's sarcoma occurring in Europe and the Americas between 1902 and 1966. All of the cases occurred in people less than 60 years old, and all of the people died within two and a half years of illness. In addition, many of the patients also had opportunistic infections. And all of these cases would meet the CDC definition of AIDS.

Katner and Pankey, based on this information, argue that HIV infection and AIDS had existed in an endemic form in Europe and the Americas at least since the beginning of the century. HIV was not recognized because of the low level of infectivity. The sexual revolution, particularly as pertaining to homosexual practices, and the drug culture caused the epidemic. The virus was subsequently introduced into Africa; however, the authors did not discuss how HIV was introduced into Africa.

I had held the same view that the AIDS epidemic started from the "West" and was later introduced into Africa but I was not sure how it occurred. During the Fourth International Conference in Stockholm, I was talking with a delegate from Nigeria and asked him what he thought was the reason that Nigeria, with more than 100 million in population, had fewer than 10 reported cases of AIDS. His response was that it might have to do with tourism. Travel would spread the disease but tourism was not big in Nigeria. Since the conversation with the Nigerian delegate, I have taken a closer look at the African countries with the largest number of AIDS cases—and I have concluded that European tourists introduced HIV into Africa.

It has often been said that the African countries that were colonized by France did not gain real independence because many of them retained a lot of French culture and close political and economic ties with France. Similar relationships have existed between Belgium and her former African colonies. On the other hand, former British colonies cut most ties with Britain after independence. An effect of the French and Belgian influence is frequent travel between these European countries and the former colonies by nationals of both continents. Also, many French and Belgian nationals live and work in former African colonies. These Europeans tend to have close interaction with African nationals.

The so-called African AIDS belt comprises Zaire, Rwanda, Burundi, Uganda, Tanzania, Central African Republic, and Zambia—all in Central and East Africa. There is evidence that AIDS spread from Central Africa (Zaire, Rwanda, Burundi) to East Africa by the

Rwanda-Uganda-Kenya Highway. In West Africa, only the Côte d'Ivoire and Ghana have more than 1,000 reported cases of AIDS. Konotey-Ahulu reported that all but 2 of the 145 cases of AIDS in Ghana by 1987 were in Ghanaian prostitutes who had been working in the Côte d'Ivoire; they contracted the disease there and had been sent home to die. The other two cases were a Ghanaian man and his German wife; the couple had previously lived in Germany for 15 years. In other words, all reported cases of AIDS in Ghana up to 1987 resulted from contraction of HIV outside the country, making the Côte d'Ivoire the only country in West Africa with a major HIV-infection problem in the early to mid-1980s.

The Côte d'Ivoire has had a relatively stable and prosperous economy since independence from France in 1960. This stability has been attriubted to the close political and economic ties between the Côte d'Ivoire and France. Many French businessmen and other experts stayed in the Côte d'Ivoire after independence, contributing to its economic stability. The strong French presence in the Côte d'Ivoire involves a lot of travel to and from France. On the other hand, Ghana's economy has undergone turmoil since the early 1970s. The Côte d'Ivoire became a place for many Ghanaians to go for work. Some of the Ghanaian women working in the Côte d'Ivoire indulged in prostitution to supplement their incomes; others engaged in prostitution full time. Their clients included native Ivorians and foreign nationals. There is a lot of traveling by the Ghanaian residents of the Côte d'Ivoire back and forth to Ghana.

French and Belgian nationals are similarly present in the Central African countries of Zaire, Congo, Rwanda, and Burundi. And there is a lot of travel between those countries and Europe. There also is a lot of travel between those countries and East African countries, particularly those in the African AIDS belt.

I propose that there are two foci of the original HIV infection/AIDS in Africa: the Côte d'Ivoire and Central Africa (Zaire, Congo, Rwanda, Burundi), that HIV was introduced to the two foci from Europe, and that the introduction was through the close ties between those foci and certain European countries. From the two foci, HIV/AIDS spread to other countries. The spread was through travel and tourism, and prostitution played a major role in the spread, as discussed in the case of the Côte d'Ivoire. And the spread from Central Africa to East Africa through prostitutes and truck drivers on the Rwanda-Uganda-Kenya Highway is well documented.

## MISCONCEPTIONS ABOUT AFRICAN AIDS

In this chapter, I have tried to discuss the situation in Africa regarding AIDS and HIV infection. The aim is to dispel or clarify some rather widespread misconceptions or views about AIDS in Africa. The discussion has been on two major points: (a) AIDS in Africa is different than that in other parts of the world. (b) AIDS originated in Africa. The conclusion is that both viewpoints are false. Because the discussion was rather long, I believe a summary is in order.

### African AIDS Is Different

The major reason for this view is the 1:1 male-to-female ratio of AIDS cases in Africa. It has been concluded that the ratio is due to the heterosexual transmission of HIV, whereas homosexual transmission is the reason for the 13:1 ratio in the United States and Europe. Because there is relatively less heterosexual transmission in the West, it was thought that there may be something unique or different about heterosexual activity by Africans. I maintain that other factors such as genital ulcers and other STDs, blood transfusion, and medical injections contribute to this ratio. Furthermore, non-Africans residing in African countries with high numbers of AIDS cases have a similar ratio. A study reported in the *British Medical Journal* (Bonneaux, 1988) found the male-to-female ratio of AIDS cases among Belgians living in certain African countries to be 2.3:1—much closer to "African AIDS" than to "European AIDS." Bonneaux and his coworkers also tested Belgians who had lived in Africa for HIV antibodies. They found those who tested positive to have been involved in or subjected to the same practices as Africans. That is, they had had more heterosexual contact with Africans, had received blood transfusions, and had gotten medical injections by untrained personnel. The more than 1,400 Belgians in the study were living or had lived in Rwanda, Burundi, or Zaire. The study supports the idea that there is nothing unique about heterosexual activity by Africans that puts them at greater risk for acquiring HIV. Neither is there anything unique about their genetic makeup.

Other "evidence" that African AIDS is different is the clinical presentation of most African AIDS patients. African AIDS patients tend to have dermatological and diarrheal illnesses more often, whereas AIDS patients in the United States and Europe tend to have generalized lymphadenopathy and pneumonia. Cryptosporidiosis, crypto-coccal meningitis, and herpes simplex virus infections are more common in African AIDS patients, whereas 63% of U.S. and European AIDS patients have *Pneumocystis carinii* pneumonia. This is really a reflection of an association between endemic diseases and AIDS. The basic definition of AIDS is the destruction of the body's immune system so that a person becomes subjected to common and unusual infections. It makes sense that a person with AIDS would develop common and unusual infection endemic to his or her area of residence. So the different clinical manifestations mentioned above are not a reason to declare African AIDS different; to say otherwise indicates lack of understanding of the disease process.

## AIDS Is Killing Millions of Africans

As clearly discussed, AIDS is not killing millions of people in Africa *yet*; it has the potential to do so, however. Only a few countries are currently reporting high numbers of cases. Even those countries with major problems with AIDS have much higher morbidity and mortality rates for conditions such as malaria, tuberculosis, measles, and diarrheal illnesses. It has often been said that there is underreporting of AIDS cases from Africa. I maintain that, even if only 10% of cases are being reported, the true numbers would be hundreds of thousands, not millions, as is the case for the other diseases.

Indeed, there could be overreporting in some situations when the Bangui criteria (WHO, 1986) are used to identify AIDS cases. The WHO had a workshop in Bangui, Central African Republic, in 1986 and developed a provisional clinical definition of AIDS to be used for diagnosis where sophisticated diagnostic equipment is not available. In the absence of antibodies to or isolation of HIV, it can be difficult to distinguish AIDS from other illnesses when the Bangui criteria (Table 5.1) are used for the diagnosis of AIDS. For example, severe weight loss could be due to lack of adequate nutrient intake (or other respiratory infections); persistent cough could be due to tuberculosis in the absence of HIV infection; and chronic diarrhea is not uncommon in many African countries. Studies in Zaire have shown that only 59% of AIDS cases diagnosed by the Bangui criteria had HIV infection. Tuberculosis was the most common illness by which false positive diagnoses of AIDS were made with the clinical definition; TB gives many of the same signs as used in the Bangui clinical definition of AIDS.

**Table 5.1**   Provisional WHO Clinical Definition of AIDS

Adults:

AIDS in an adult is defined by the existence of at least two major signs associated with at least one minor sign in the absence of known causes of immunosuppression such as cancer or severe malnutrition or other recognized etiologies.

Major signs
(a)   Weight loss greater than 10% body weight
(b)   Chronic diarrhea more than 1 month
(c)   Prolonged fever more than 1 month (intermittent or constant)

Minor signs
(a)   Persistent cough for more than 1 month
(b)   Generalized pruritic dermatitis
(c)   Recurrent herpes zoster
(d)   Oropharyngeal candidiasis
(e)   Chronic progressive disseminated herpes simplex infection
(f)   Generalized lymphadenopathy

The presence of generalized Kaposi's sarcoma or cryptococcal meningitis are sufficient by themselves for the diagnosis of AIDS.

Children:

Pediatric AIDS is suspected in an infant or child presenting with at least two major signs associated with at least two minor signs in the absence of known causes of immunosuppression.

Major signs
(a)   Weight loss or abnormally slow growth
(b)   Chronic diarrhea more than 1 month
(c)   Prolonged fever more than 1 month

Minor signs
(a)   Generalized lymphadenopathy
(b)   Oropharyngeal candidiasis
(c)   Repeated common infections (otitis, pharyngitis, and so forth)
(d)   Persistent cough more than 1 month
(e)   Generalized dermatitis
(f)   Confirmed maternal LAV/HTLV-III infection

SOURCE: World Health Organization (1986).

In addition to the Bangui criteria as a possible means of overreporting, serologic tests used in some African countries may contribute to a possible overestimation of AIDS/HIV infection. Many of the tests used earlier during the epidemic were inaccurate, and much of the data published up to 1985 have been discarded. Cross-reactivity of the HIV antigen with antigens of tropical organisms, such as the organism that causes malaria, continues to be a problem in some countries. Until such time that tests for HIV are purified, the potential for overestimating the problem will continue to exist.

## AIDS Originated in Africa

The evidence for this belief includes the detection of antibodies to HIV in serum from Africans as early as late 1950s and early 1960s, and there is close similarity between SIV found in African green monkeys and HIV. The theory is that SIV got into humans in Central and East Africa where the green monkeys are most common and underwent mutation to become HIV, and then HIV was subsequently exported to America and Europe. Recent studies have found HIV antibodies in serum from Americans and Europeans during the same time periods as those found in Africans.

I have discussed the evidence that disputes the SIV-HIV connection in regard to the African green monkey. HIV has probably always existed. It had not caused an epidemic because the right conditions for an epidemic had not existed. The sexual revolution and drug culture in the United States and Europe in the late 1960s and early 1970s caused the transmission and propagation of HIV, with the subsequent epidemic in the early 1980s. HIV/AIDS was subsequently introduced to the Côte d'Ivoire and a few Central African countries and spread to other African countries.

The reason AIDS has taken a rather quick foothold in certain African countries is that the right environment existed before the introduction of HIV/AIDS. Genital ulcers and other STDs, blood transfusions, and medical injections were common and facilitated transmission of HIV and the development of AIDS. Prostitutes and truck drivers have been the means of transmission of AIDS within and between countries. Dawson (1988) has asked why there is a higher prevalence of genital ulcers and other STDs in many African countries than in the West. He takes a historical perspective in responding to this question, particularly the role of prostitution.

Dawson uses Kenya as a prototype country in discussing how urbanization effected the spread of syphilis. European colonial authorities had large agricultural estates and small industries for which cheap African labor was needed. In the early 1920s, a large number of African men migrated to these areas, and the influx increased in the

1940s as towns became larger and urbanized. These men usually went to take temporary work that lasted for lengthy periods and left their families behind. Long absence from wives, or, for unmarried men, no wives, attracted the working men to prostitutes for female companionship. The same urbanization process drew women to the developing cities; the women had few employment opportunities and found prostitution a rather lucrative alternative.

The multiple sexual partners involved in prostitution led to the propagation of syphilis in these urban and other labor-intensive centers. Working men and women from these centers traveled to their hometowns quite often and thereby introduced syphilis to the rural areas of Kenya. Meanwhile, new industries in the urban areas required effective rail and road transportation; railway stations and lorry (truck) stops became centers of prostitution and contributed to the spread of syphilis.

Syphilis did not spread quickly in rural Kenya in the 1920s and 1930s because of the prevalence of yaws disease, which provided cross-immunity to syphilis. Syphilis started spreading in the 1940s after colonial medical officials had conducted an extensive anti-yaws campaign, which essentially removed the immunity that yaws had provided against syphilis. Unfortunately, the use of heavy-metal chemotherapy did not cure yaws; it suppressed the symptoms but succeeded in preventing a generation of children from growing up with potential immunity to syphilis.

So the colonial administrative practice of using migrant labor effected the dismantling of families, the establishment and perpetuation of prostitution, and the spread of syphilis. Kenya's history is common to that of many African countries, particularly countries in East and Central Africa. The spread of syphilis was accompanied by other STDs. Many of these diseases could have been easily treated, but poverty and lack of access to adequate medical care promoted the perpetuation of the STDs. Therefore, genital lesions and other STDs remained strong in these countries during the colonial period.

After independence, many of these countries continued colonial practices. Migrant labor remained prominent in the increasing urbanization. Though employment opportunities improved for women, jobs have remained relatively fewer for them and the pay often small. Prostitution has remained quite lucrative. In addition to the strong labor migration from one's own hometown or region, prostitution has been supported by tourism—a postindependence industry for many of these countries. Migrant workers (and prostitutes) travel within and between countries.

Thus, when HIV was introduced into Africa in the early 1980s, the right conditions—conditions having origins in and in existence from the colonial period—were present for its rather fast spread. The same migrant labor/prostitution pattern, travel within and between countries, and tourism that promoted the spread of syphilis and other STDs has caused the spread of HIV infection. The pattern of poverty and lack of access to adequate medical care exist in the AIDS era. Therefore, not only has HIV spread quickly but also the progression to AIDS has been rather quick.

## REFERENCES

AIDS in Africa. (1989, July 25). *Lancet*, pp. 192-194.

AIDS: The year in review. (1988). *Internal Medicine World Report, 3*, 29-38.

Biggar, R. T., et al. (1985). ELISA: HLTV antibody reactivity associated with malaria and immune complexes in healthy Africans. *Lancet, 2*, 520-523.

Bryant, M. L., et al. (1985). Molecular comparison of retroviruses associated with human and simian AIDS. *Hematology and Oncology, 3*, 187-197.

Clumeck, N. (1986). Epidemiological correlations between African AIDS and AIDS in Europe. *Infection, 14*, 97-99.

Clumeck, N., et al. (1985). Seroepidemiological studies of HTLV-III antibody prevalence among selected groups of heterosexual Africans. *JAMA, 254*, 2591-2602.

Dawson, M. H. (1988). AIDS in Africa: Historical roots. In N. Miller & R. C. Rockwell (Eds.), *AIDS in Africa: The social and policy impact*. Lewiston/Queenston: Edwin Mellen.

Hag, C. (1988). Data on AIDS in Africa: An assessment. In N. Miller & R. C. Rockwell (Eds.), *AIDS in Africa: The social and policy impact*. Lewiston/Queenston: Edwin Mellen.

Kanki, P. J., et al. (1985). Isolation of T-lymphotropic virus related to HTLV-III/LAV from wild caught African monkeys. *Science, 230*, 951-954.

Katner, H. P., & Pankey, G. A. (1987). Evidence for a Euro-American origin of human immunodeficiency virus (HIV). *Journal of the National Medical Association, 79*, 1069-1072.

Konotey-Ahulu, F. I. D. (1987a, May 30). Group-specific component and HIV infection. *Lancet*, p. 1287.

Konotey-Ahulu, F. I. D. (1987b, July 25). AIDS in Africa: Misinformation and disinformation. *Lancet*, pp. 206-207.

Kreiss, J. K., et al. (1986). AIDS virus infections in Nairobi prostitutes. *The New England Journal of Medicine, 314*, 414-418.

Marlink, R. G., & Essex, M. (1987). Africa and the biology of HIV infection. *JAMA, 257*, 2632-2633.

Miller, N., & Rockwell, R. C. (Eds.). (1988). *AIDS in Africa: The social and policy impact.* Lewiston/Queenston: Edwin Mellen.

Nahmias, S. J., et al. (1986). Evidence for human infection with HTLV-III/LAV-like virus in Central Africa, 1959. *Lancet, 1,* 1214-1216.

Nzibambi, N. (1988). The prevalence of infection with human immunodeficiency virus over a 10-year period in rural Zaire. *The New England Journal of Medicine, 318,* 276-279.

Piot, P., et al. (1987). Retrospective seroepidemiology of AIDS virus infection in Nairobi populations. *Journal of Infectious Disease, 115,* 1108-1112.

Quinn, T. C., et al. (1986). Aids in Africa: An epidemiologic paradigm. *Science, 234,* 955-963.

Quinn, T. C., et al. (1987). Serologic and immunologic studies in patients with AIDS in North America and Africa: The potential role of infectious agents as cofactors in human immunodeficiency virus infection. *JAMA, 257,* 2617-2621.

Tortey, B., et al. (1988). Epidemiology of HIV and AIDS in Africa: Emerging issues and social implications. In N. Miller & R. C. Rockwell (Eds.), *AIDS in Africa: The social and policy impact.* Lewiston/Queenston: Edwin Mellen.

Williamson, W. A., & Greenwood, B. M. (1978). Impairment of immune response to vaccination after acute malaria. *Lancet, 1,* 1328-1329.

World Health Organization. (1986). WHO Workshop on AIDS in Central Africa. *Weekly Epidemiology Research, 61,* 72-73.

# 6

# AIDS and HIV Infection: Genetics Versus the Environment

The central issue, the *raîson d'être,* of this book is the role of genes in acquisition of HIV and/or progression to AIDS. The question of genes is raised because of several reports making an association between race/ethnicity and HIV infection. There is a disproportionately high rate of AIDS in black Americans; HIV infection has spread rather quickly in several black African countries; and several serologic studies have demonstrated a higher HIV-antibody status in blacks than in other populations. These trends have led to the question of whether there is something *different* about black people in terms of their susceptibility to HIV infection.

A hint about a racial association with AIDS first originated because of Haitians living in the United States during the early part of the AIDS epidemic. When epidemiologists met to categorize AIDS cases reported to the CDC, several risk factors were identified. There were quite a large number of AIDS cases among Haitian residents in the United States. In addition to its prevalence among Haitians, these victims seemed to have none of the recognized risk factors—homosexual activity, IV drug use, or blood transfusion. Being Haitian (black) then became a risk factor on its own for AIDS.

The epidemiological data on AIDS prevalence in blacks are well established. As detailed in earlier chapters of this book, black Americans have the highest rate of AIDS and HIV infection among all U.S. racial/ethnic groups. High rates exist for black Americans for both males and females, for all age groups, and in all risk categories except hemophiliacs. The high rates among U.S. blacks exist in all the major geographic areas of the United States. And these trends have remained relatively constant over the years.

There has been speculation that AIDS in Africa is different than that in other parts of the world because of its so-called heterosexual transmission, different clinical presentation, and the speed with which the disease has spread in many African countries. Furthermore, it is supposed that AIDS is killing millions of Africans. The issue of AIDS in Africa has been thoroughly discussed in the last chapter—with the conclusion that it is no different. Yet the prevalence of AIDS among black Africans, black Americans, and Haitians understandably leads to the question of more susceptibility to HIV infection and the development of AIDS by black people. The question is really twofold: (a) Are blacks really more susceptible to HIV infection and AIDS? (b) Why are they more susceptible than other racial/ethnic groups?

As discussed earlier in this and other chapters, there are many reports that make an association between black race and HIV infection/AIDS. These reports have led to the widely accepted notion that being black is a risk factor for AIDS (which will be discussed in more depth later). The main question then is why blacks are more susceptible. More studies on this issue have been conducted with black Americans. The "clearest" identifying factor is IV drug use. Blacks represent the highest proportion of U.S. cases of AIDS contracted through IV drug use, therefore, IV drug use has been accepted by many as *the* reason for the prevalence of AIDS among blacks. If this were the case, how does one explain its prevalence in black Africans and Haitians? In addition, how does one explain the highest rates for black Americans in all risk categories of AIDS? The logical conclusion is that there is (or there may be) something genetically different about black people that makes them more susceptible to HIV infection.

## POSSIBLE GENETIC MARKERS FOR SUSCEPTIBILITY TO HIV INFECTION

There are many reports in the medical literature on the association between genetic markers and both human and animal disease. Genetic markers may be protective or destructive; that is, the marker may provide the host with resistance to a disease or lead to susceptibility to a disease. The important thing about these markers is that their presence involves an association between them and certain diseases and does not necessarily involve a direct relationship of cause and effect.

Perhaps the most well-studied association between a genetic marker and resistance to disease is that between the sickle-cell gene and malaria. A mutation in normal hemoglobin (HbA) produces an abnormal hemoglobin (HbS) that leads to "sickling" of red blood cells under certain circumstances. Individuals who are homozygous—that is, who carry two copies of HbS—have sickle-cell disease; they suffer from frequent "crises" and often die at a young age. Individuals who are heterozygous—that is, who possess only one copy of HbS—have sickle-cell trait. They are usually healthy and live a normal life span.

The significant thing about sickle-cell trait is an apparent resistance to malaria. Many reports have demonstrated a lower prevalence of malaria among individuals heterozygous for HbS (i.e., AS) than among both those homozygous for HbS (i.e., SS) and those with normal hemoglobin (i.e., AA). The indication is that the HbS provides an inhospitable environment to the *Plasmodium falciparum* (the causative agent of malaria) because of low oxygen tension in deep tissues where the *Plasmodia* mature.

An example of genetic markers and susceptibility to disease is the group of markers called the *human leukocyte antigen* (HLA) complex. It is a multigene complex associated with many diseases. The best known example is the association of HLA with ankylosing spondylitis. Ankylosing spondylitis is a chronic progressive form of arthritis characterized by inflammation and stiffness of the spine. It usually affects young males aged 10 to 30. Individuals possessing HLA-B27 are about 300 times more likely than those without it to acquire ankylosing spondylitis; and about 90% of individuals with ankylosing spondylitis possess HLA-B27. Indeed, HLA-B27 is so common in ankylosing spondylitis that testing for the gene complex is part of the diagnostic work-up for the disease.

It is important to bear in mind that the relationships between genetic markers and disease, whether of resistance or susceptibility, is one of association and not cause and effect. Indeed, Konotey-Ahulu (1972) has challenged the claim that HbS in the heterozygous state provides resistance to falciparum malaria. He offers the theory of *balanced polymorphism* to explain his claim (Konotey-Ahulu, 1972). There is no *proof* that HbS *causes* resistance to falciparum malaria, nor is there *proof* that HLA-B27 *causes* susceptibility to ankylosing spondylitis. But the associations appear strong enough for widespread acceptance. Associations between genetic markers and AIDS have been reported.

An association between HLA and AIDS has been identified in at least two clinical situations. HLA-DR5 has been found in high rates in patients with Kaposi's sarcoma; about 60% of Kaposi's sarcoma patients in one study expressed the HLA-DR5 gene, whereas only 21% of controls expressed it. There is also an association of HLA-B35 with progression from persistent generalized lymphadenopathy (PGL) to AIDS. A study reported by Scorza-Smeraldi and others found that 76% of patients with PGL who progressed to AIDS possessed HLA-B35, whereas 29% of healthy controls and 29% of PGL patients without progression to AIDS possessed the gene (Scorza-Smeraldi et al., 1986).

Perhaps the best known and most controversial findings on the association between genetic markers and AIDS is the one reported by Eales et al. (1987). Their study involved the genetic factor known as group specific component (Gc). The Gc gene has several alleles, and, according to the Eales group, possession of one allele may be protective whereas possession of another allele of the same gene may enhance progression to AIDS (Eales et al., 1987).

The Gc gene is a glycoprotein found on cells and in serum. It possesses three alleles that are distinct in terms of electrophoretic mobility; Gc1 fast (Gc1f), Gc1 slow (Gc1s), and Gc2. The Gc phenotype is distributed in populations by classical Mendelian inheritance; that is, an individual may be homozygous or heterozygous. Gc is required for vitamin D binding and metabolism; it is known to effect transport of large amounts of calcium through binding to vitamin D.

The Eales group studied a group of white homosexual males in London. The study group included AIDS patients, their HIV-negative sexual partners, HIV-positive individuals without symptoms, individuals with persistent generalized lymphadenopathy (PGL), and ARC patients. Seronegative homosexuals and heterosexuals were used as controls. The study involved the distribution of the different alleles of Gc in the study population. The following were the major findings: (a) AIDS patients had a higher frequency of Gc1f than controls—53.2% versus 17.6%. (b) AIDS patients had a lower frequency of Gc2 than controls—18.3% versus 28.7%. (c) More AIDS patients were homozygous for Gc1f than controls—30.2% versus 0.8%. (d) There was a strong positive association between severity of clinical symptoms and Gc1f but a negative association between clinical symptoms and Gc2. The conclusion is that Gc1f may enhance progression to AIDS whereas Gc2 may be protective.

Subsequent to the report by Eales et al., Giles et al. (1987) reported their study of white homosexual men in San Francisco. That study used an experimental design similar to that of Eales to assess the frequency of different Gc alleles and the association between the alleles and AIDS. They found no association between any Gc allele and susceptibility or resistance to HIV infection or progression to AIDS. Two other studies, from Houston and from Norway (Constans, 1978a), reached the same conclusions as the Giles group. Finally, Papiha (1987) has disputed the Eales findings on epidemiological grounds; that is, if there were indeed an association between Gc alleles and AIDS, one would expect the frequency of that allele in a population to parallel the prevalence of AIDS in that population. He presents data to the contrary (Papiha, 1987).

The study of Eales et al. that presented an association between Gc alleles and AIDS was on white male homosexuals. The investigators, however, used the data from that study to conclude that the frequency of Gc alleles in black people may explain the high prevalence of AIDS in blacks. The Eales study has been challenged on both counts; that is, there may not be an association between Gc alleles and AIDS, and the high prevalence of AIDS in blacks may not be explained by the frequency of Gc alleles.

As stated above, the study by Eales et al. involved white homosexual males in London. The other studies that disputed Eales's finding were also conducted with white homosexual males in the United States and Europe. These latter studies failed to duplicate the observation that Gc1f alleles may provide susceptibility to AIDS and Gc2 may provide resistance. The conclusion one is likely to draw from these findings should be that there may or may not be any evidence for an association between Gc alleles and AIDS in *white male homosexuals*. However, the nature of scientific investigation allows for the extrapolation of data to other situations. Hence, Eales et al. suggested a possible relationship between Gc alleles and the prevalence of AIDS in black people.

From their findings that there was a correlation between Gc1f and AIDS symptomatology, Eales et al. suggested that the Gc1f allele may promote viral (HIV) entry to cells or directly affect viral infection. By that means, they observe: "It is of interest that in an area where HIV infection is very common—namely, some parts of Central

Africa—the Gc1f allele predominates in the indigenous population"
(Eales et al., 1987, p. 1002). They used data from a 1978 study that
found a high frequency of Gc1f alleles in a group of pygmies in central Africa (Constans et al., 1978b). In another discussion, Eales et al. speculate
that the heterosexual spread of AIDS is more common in U.S. blacks,
and the progression to AIDS in blacks appears to be more rapid than that
in whites. This may be explained by the distribution of the Gc alleles
among white and black Americans: Gc1f and Gc2 for whites are 10%-
16% and 26%-31%, respectively; Gc1f and Gc2 for blacks are 67%-79%
and 8%-19%, respectively (Eales et al., 1987).

It should be recalled that Eales et al. made two significant observations: (a) There is a high frequency of Gc1f and a low frequency of
Gc2 alleles in the white homosexual males they studied. (b) There is a
positive association between Gc1f and progression to AIDS, but there
is a negative association between Gc2 and progression to AIDS. The
studies by Giles et al. (1987) in San Francisco and Daiger et al.
(1987) in Houston found a similar frequency of Gc alleles in the
white homosexual males they studied. Both studies failed to observe
an association (positive or negative) between Gc alleles and AIDS.
Therefore, there are two points of contention regarding the observations by Eales et al.: first, regarding whether there is an association
between Gc alleles and AIDS, and, second, whether the frequency
distribution of Gc alleles in blacks explains the prevalence of AIDS
in black populations.

Regarding the first point, it is the nature of scientific investigation
that new discoveries should be independently duplicated by others.
This has not occurred, yet the Eales finding has been widely quoted.
On the other hand, several reports have challenged the finding and
implied that there is no association between Gc alleles and AIDS. I
believe it is too early to completely discount the observation by Eales
et al. just as it is too early to fully accept it. In other words, more
studies need to be performed on different populations before we can
accept or reject the observation. The most one can say, I believe, is
that there is not enough evidence that Gc alleles provide susceptibility or resistance to AIDS.

The second point is also difficult to accept because of two potential
problems: (a) The reports by Giles et al. and Daiger et al. indicate that
the frequency of Gc alleles does not correlate with susceptibility or resistance to AIDS. This implies that the frequency of Gc alleles (high
Gc1f and low Gc2) in blacks may not correlate with their susceptibility

to AIDS. (b) Even if the frequency of the Gc allele clearly correlated with susceptibility in the reported studies (in white homosexual males), no such observation has been made in blacks. Yet, most of the discussion concerning genetic susceptibility and AIDS has been focused on blacks; that is, there appears to be a widespread perception that the prevalence of AIDS in blacks may be due to their genetic susceptibility to the disease.

Obviously, no firm conclusions can, or have been, drawn on the genetic susceptibility of blacks to AIDS. Eales et al. reported the high frequency of the Gc1f allele in blacks in Central Africa and blacks in the United States and suggested a relationship between that frequency and susceptibility to AIDS—but what was made as an "intelligent guess" has been interpreted by others as "proof." Konotey-Ahulu has accused the Eales group of implying that there is something genetically wrong with central Africans in terms of AIDS (Konotey-Ahulu, 1987). Obviously, Eales et al. did not mean that there is something genetically wrong with black people, but the comment by Dr. Konotey-Ahulu illustrates the problems involved in interpreting scientific reports.

In Chapter 1, I referred to a publication by the Harris County Medical Society. The booklet is titled *AIDS: A Guide for Survival* and it has very good information on AIDS in lay terminology. More than a million copies of the booklet have been distributed in Texas. Reference is made to the reports by Eales et al. and Daiger et al. regarding genetic susceptibility to AIDS. The booklet concludes:

> Variations in these genes found in different populations could also explain why the AIDS virus has spread so quickly in Central Africa and why the percentage of blacks with AIDS in the United States is disproportionate . . . the Gc1 fast gene that seems to increase susceptibility is found more frequently in African blacks than in Caucasians. (Harris County Medical Society, 1987, p. 42)

During presentations on AIDS throughout Texas, I have often been asked about blacks' potential genetic susceptibility to AIDS. Most of the questioners refer to the booklet and frame their questions in a manner that suggests there is no doubt about it. In other words, there is such a high rate of AIDS among blacks because they possess a gene that makes them more susceptible to the disease. The authors clearly did not intend to pass on the information as facts proved beyond reasonable doubt. But that is how many members of the public have perceived it.

There is no question that the connection between Gc alleles and the prevalence of AIDS in blacks is a tenuous one. Until such time that biochemical studies have been done in different black populations to document the correlation between the Gc alleles and progression to AIDS, the connection should be regarded only as a *possibility*. Caution should be exercised in discussing the issue to prevent leaving a false impression either way. Research must continue on the gene issue as well as on other possibilities. Research on why there is such a high rate of AIDS in blacks should obviously not be limited to the genetic aspects; other factors should also be investigated. For example, what role does the environment play in susceptibility of AIDS?

The discussion in this chapter so far has concerned the possible link between genetic markers and AIDS. There appears to be a possible link through the human leukocyte antigen (HLA) complex and the group specific component (Gc) genes. Studies on both markers have not been done specifically with black people. Yet data from Gc studies have been extrapolated to explain the high prevalence of AIDS in blacks. This and other information has led to the widespread conception that blacks are more susceptible to HIV infection and progression to AIDS.

The notion of *susceptibility,* particularly if the word is preceded by *genetic,* implies uniqueness. Therefore, if a group of people or a particular population has genetic susceptibility, then there is something unique, something innate, about that population that produces the susceptibility. It is in this context that many people view blacks' potential susceptibility to AIDS. In other words, being black is a risk on its own in acquiring the disease. As discussed in this chapter, there is no conclusive evidence that blacks are genetically susceptible to AIDS. Indeed, it is questionable that blacks are truly more susceptible. They do not have the highest number of AIDS cases; they do have a *disproportionately high* rate based on their population. If they are more susceptible, I contend that there is an environmental instead of genetic susceptibility.

## GENETIC VERSUS ENVIRONMENTAL SUSCEPTIBILITY TO DISEASE

Human beings exist—we are born, we grow, and we die—through a dynamic interaction between our genetic makeup and environmental conditions. Genetic makeup is established at conception. A person's growth and development depend upon the interaction between genetic and environmental factors right after conception. The environmental factors are both internal and external; and the dynamic interaction starting at conception continues after birth through to death. The genetic makeup stays relatively constant, whereas environmental conditions change during a person's life span.

A person's health results from the dynamic interaction between his or her genetic makeup and the environmental conditions to which he or she is subjected. Disease may result from this dynamic interplay. Thus most diseases probably have some genetic component, although there are purely "genetic" diseases and purely "environmental" diseases. For example, bacterial infections are considered purely environmental diseases, but males tend to be slightly more susceptible to them than females.

*Genes* are molecules of deoxyribonucleic acid (DNA) that are carried on chromosomes. Genes are the basic unit of heredity, and each of the 46 chromosomes possessed by each human being has thousands of genes. Genetic disease results from defects in a gene or a group of genes or from chromosomal abnormalities. Defects in genes may result from a single-gene mutation or several gene defects; chromosomal abnormalities may result from structural defects or deviations from the normal number of chromosomes.

Because the gene is the basic unit of heredity, purely genetic diseases are inherited. They are acquired during pregnancy, and the individual born with such a genetic disease has no choice but to develop symptoms of the disease after birth. All individuals born with the gene defect or chromosomal abnormality have the same disease with the characteristic symptomatology. Sickle-cell anemia is an example of a purely genetic disease resulting from a single gene mutation. Occurring mostly in black people, individuals born with the defect all have "sickling" of red blood cells and its attendant symptoms. Down's syndrome (Mongolism) is an example of a purely genetic disease resulting from chromosomal abnormality. Individuals with the condition are born with an extra chromosome 21, and they have the characteristic facies and other problems like mental retardation.

In addition to the purely genetic diseases, there are other genetic diseases that involve associations. These may be genetic markers that interact with other nongenetic factors to produce a disease or group of diseases. These are not purely genetic diseases, and affected individuals may have different degrees or different symptoms of the disease. Examples of genetic markers and various diseases have been given earlier in the chapter. A third type of genetic disease is one without a clearly recognized gene or chromosomal defect or a genetic marker but that appears to be inherited. Such diseases are often referred to as "running in families." They seem to be passed on from parents to offspring. Breast cancer occurs more often in daughters whose mothers had had the disease than in the general population, although there is no clearly identified genetic defect for the disease. Similarly, alcoholism seems to run in families.

One of the fascinating things about science and medicine is that issues are seldom "black and white"; they are often "grey." Therefore, there is really no such thing as a *purely* genetic disease. For example, two individuals born with sickle cell may not have the same characteristics. They may have exactly the same gene mutation and may both be homozygous. However, the degree of anemia, the number and frequency of crises, and their life spans may be different. These may depend upon where they live and their economic status, nutritional status, and emotional stress. So, a "purely" genetic disease like sickle-cell disease may not be so pure. The extent of disability from a genetic defect depends a lot upon environmental conditions. It is conceivable that a genetic defect may not lead to any illness or disability if the right environmental conditions do not exist.

I often use alcoholism as an example of a possible genetic defect with no consequent disability. There is controversy over whether alcoholism is a disease. There is even more disagreement over whether it is a genetic disease. Some believe it is genetic because of its prevalence in some families and certain population groups. And there may be genetic markers for susceptibility to alcoholism.

Suppose alcoholism is a purely genetic disease—that is, that there is a gene defect that makes individuals born with the defect susceptible to alcoholism. An individual with the defective gene must be exposed to alcohol to develop alcoholism. Suppose such an individual is born and lives in a country where alcohol consumption is not permitted by law (as in Saudi Arabia). If this individual lives all his life in that country and is never exposed to alcohol, he will not develop the disease called alcoholism. The genetic defect, if it existed, would be meaningless in this case. This means that a genetic defect requires the right environmental conditions in some cases to be expressed in the form of an illness or disability.

I view the genetic susceptibility of blacks to AIDS in a similar manner as alcoholism. First, there is no proof of a genetic susceptibility. Second, I submit that it would be meaningless, it would not be expressed, unless the right environmental conditions existed. In other words, like alcoholism, the environment plays a more prominent role than genetics in terms of the prevalence of AIDS in black people. And the environment includes the health care system to which many black people have been subjected.

## Epidemiology

A lot of the knowledge on AIDS has been obtained from epidemiological studies. Indeed, epidemiology is indispensable to the understanding of a new disease, particularly one with the pandemic distribution of AIDS. The use of epidemiology has led to the understanding and better control of many diseases in history.

*Epidemiology* may be defined as the study of the *distribution* and *determinants* of diseases and injuries in human populations. The way diseases are distributed and the factors that influence the distribution (determinants) can lead to intelligent guesses about the nature of a particular disease. The implication from the definition of epidemiology is that diseases are unevenly distributed in populations, and the uneven distribution can be a basis for concluding causal relationships between certain population characteristics and diseases. Morris (1955, p. 395) put it this way:

> The main function of epidemiology is to discover groups in the population with high rates of diseases, and with low, so that causes of disease and of freedom from disease can be postulated. . . . The biggest promise of this method lies in relating diseases to the ways of living of different groups, and by doing so to unravel "causes" of disease *about which it is possible to do something* [italics added].

The significance of the above quotation is the use of epidemiological studies to find causes of diseases about which something can be done. The implication is that there may not be a need to find the true "scientific" cause of a disease in order to control it. Modification of certain factors influencing the cause and/or severity of the disease may lead to adequate or even complete control of a disease. A classic

example of this phenomenon is John Snow and the water pumps involved in a cholera epidemic in London.

An outbreak of cholera was killing hundreds of people in London
in 1853. As scientists struggled to find the cause of the epidemic and
ways to control it, John Snow, a London physician, made a simple
suggestion—turn off the water pumps supplying water to the neighborhoods with the highest numbers of deaths from cholera. This was
done, and the epidemic was brought under control. The epidemic was
controlled without knowing the cause of cholera; Snow accomplished
his feat about 30 years before Koch discovered *Vibrio cholerae* to be
the causative agent of cholera.

Snow used epidemiological principles to study the cholera epidemic and came to the conclusion that cholera might be transmitted
by discharge of fecal material into water supplies. He investigated the
water supply for each household where a fatal cholera attack had occurred. His figures demonstrated that most deaths were occurring in
the neighborhoods supplied by one company, the Southwark and
Vauxhall Company; the lowest number of deaths was in areas supplied by another company, the Lambeth Company. It turned out that
the Southwark and Vauxhall Company drew its water from the
Thames River downstream, where the water had been contaminated
by waste. The Lambeth Company drew water upstream, where the
water was free of contamination. Snow's analysis of death rates
showed a 20:1 ratio between areas supplied by the two companies,
that is, individuals living in households supplied by Southwark and
Vauxhall (contaminated water) were dying 20 times more frequently
than those supplied by Lambeth.

The significance of the Snow story above is the fact that Dr. Snow
focused his attention on the aspect of the epidemic *about which something could be done*. Something was done based on his findings, and
the epidemic was controlled—30 years before the causative agent of
cholera was discovered. It is interesting to note that, with knowledge
of the causative agent and effective antibiotics to treat it, personal hygiene (originating from Snow's idea) is still the recommended approach to controlling cholera infections and epidemics. Washing
hands meticulously, boiling water before drinking or using it to pre-
pare food, and controlling flies are extremely effective in controlling
cholera transmission even today. These measures do not require
knowledge of the causative agent or the pathogenesis of cholera. In
addition, they are more practical, simpler, and cheaper to implement.

I have told the story about John Snow and the cholera epidemic to make a point, which is that we need to apply more epidemiology to the AIDS epidemic. We should do this by applying Morris's definition of epidemiology, that is, trying to focus more attention on the aspects of AIDS about which something can be done. In this regard, I believe we should not spend too much time and resources on arguing whether blacks are genetically more susceptible to AIDS. Instead, we should pay more attention to the epidemiology of AIDS vis-á-vis black people; we should take an ecological view of AIDS in blacks and thereby try to find some things about which we can do something.

Proof of a clear genetic susceptibility to AIDS would be a good thing. It would add to the understanding of this devastating disease. But it is likely to have limited usefulness as individual black AIDS patients and the black population as a whole are concerned. Most genetic diseases are incurable, and treatment of such diseases is usually directed toward aspects of the disease other than the genetic ones. So knowing that a genetic marker makes blacks more susceptible is not likely to lead to better treatment or to control of the spread of the disease in that population. Indeed, it may do the opposite. As stated in Chapter 1, there could be the tendency to say that "there is nothing much to be done about it because they were born with it."

*Ecology* is defined as the study of relationships between living organisms and the environment in which they live (Last, 1983). The relationships affect health in that environmental factors impinge on the living organism and vice versa. In this regard, there is no such thing as healthy people living in an unhealthy environment—that is, an unhealthy environment may cause disease. And *environment* means the biological, physical, and social environment.

An ecological view of a disease involves consideration of the natural history of the disease. *Natural history* means the course of the disease—what happens to individuals from the point of contraction to the end of the disease process, unaffected by treatment. Without treatment, a disease may end in full recovery, temporary or permanent disability, or death. Which end product of disease is realized depends a lot upon the ecosystem, the individual, and the environment. This is because the natural history of a disease is a continuum that begins before the individual is exposed to a causal agent (see Figure 6.1).

Susceptibility is obviously the most important stage in this continuum. It is the stage before exposure to a causative agent. After exposure, however, susceptibility determines the progression through

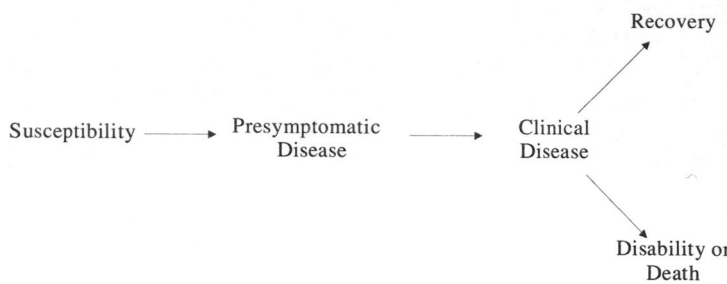

**Figure 6.1.** Disease History

the continuum. The presymptomatic disease stage occurs when the individual has been exposed to the causative agent. If the agent is an infectious one, it is the stage when infection has taken place, when the organism has "set up housekeeping" in the host. The organism reproduces itself and thereby causes tissue and/or organ damage. As tissue destruction progresses, the host may display characteristic symptoms, and signs of the particular disease are manifested—the clinical disease stage is reached. The clinical disease stage may end in complete recovery, disability, or death.

Susceptibility is determined by individual (host) factors and environmental factors (biological, physical, and social). It is related to another epidemiological principle called the "epidemiological triangle" (Figure 6.2). The triangle implies a dynamic relationship among the three components. The dynamic equilibrium may be changed and thereby influence a disease's progression (positively or negatively) if there is significant change in any of the components.

Changes in the host involve intrinsic factors that may be genetic as well as environmental factors inside the host. Genetic factors were described earlier in this chapter. Environmental factors inside the host may be existing infectious and other diseases, immunological status, and nutritional status. Environmental factors outside the host (as depicted in the epidemiological triangle) may be biological (such as plants and animals for food), physical (such as chemical pollutants), and social (such as education and housing). The intrinsic factors of the host are influenced by outside environmental factors. When the dynamic equilibrium between the host and the environment is disturbed,

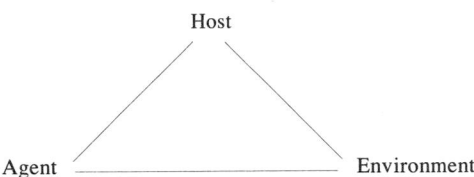

**Figure 6.2.** Epidemiological Triangle

the host may then be susceptible to the agent. But the host must be exposed to the agent before infection can occur (the presymptomatic disease stage). Whether there is progression to symptomatic disease and death or recovery depends upon the dose and virulence of the agent versus the host factors. (Recall the "dam theory.")

Regarding AIDS in black people, HIV is the agent. Host factors may be genetic and environmental inside the host; but I contend that genetic factors make little if any contribution. Environmental factors outside the host are mostly social. So, intrinsic environmental factors under the influence of extrinsic environmental factors make black people susceptible to HIV infection and quick progression to AIDS. And these are factors *about which something can be done*.

## ENVIRONMENTAL SUSCEPTIBILITY OF BLACKS TO HIV INFECTION AND AIDS

As stated earlier, most of the studies on susceptibility of blacks to AIDS have been epidemiological. These prevalence and incidence studies in various black populations have found higher rates of AIDS and HIV infection and faster progression to AIDS. These higher rates have led to the suggestion that blacks are more susceptible. And susceptibility seems to imply genetic proneness, although no studies at the biochemical level have conclusively found blacks to be genetically more susceptible to AIDS. The study by Eales et al., discussed in detail earlier in this chapter, suggests such genetic susceptibility in blacks. This may be the case, but I believe environmental factors far outweigh any possible genetic factors.

I subscribe to the environmental belief because of the distribution of AIDS in black populations. There are clear differences in prevalence of AIDS/HIV infection in blacks in different geographic areas and by socioeconomic status. A genetic disease normally does not have such an uneven distribution. For example, sickle-cell disease exists in all black populations regardless of place of residence and socioeconomic status.

In the United States, the rate of AIDS in blacks is much higher in the northeastern states such as New York and New Jersey than it is in California. Within states, it is higher in certain cities than in other cities. And, within cities, it is higher in the inner city than in suburbs and rural areas. Also, in many states, cities, and different parts of certain cities, disproportionately higher rates in blacks do not exist. In addition, regardless of state or region, AIDS in blacks is predominantly in the poor, less educated, less employed members of that race.

A similar distribution of AIDS/HIV infection exists in African blacks. It is higher in certain regions of the continent than in others. It is higher in metropolitan areas than in rural areas. And there is a demonstrated correlation between prevalence and socioeconomic status. For example, most cases of AIDS in Ghana have been in prostitutes. In Kenya, there are two classes of prostitutes: those who cater to less well-to-do men and those catering to tourists, traveling businessmen, and the wealthy elite. The prevalence of HIV infection is higher in the former group than in the latter group. In a study among hospital personnel in Zambia, the prevalence of HIV infection was found to be lowest in doctors, next lowest in medical students, and highest in nonmedical personnel.

Differences in the distribution of AIDS/HIV infection among blacks suggest that environmental rather than genetic factors may contribute to the higher prevalence in blacks. But blacks, at least U.S. blacks, are disproportionately represented by all risk categories of HIV acquisition. What environmental factors effect susceptibility to HIV infection in these risk groups?

## IV Drug Users

Of all cases of AIDS in U.S. blacks, 39% were attributed to IV drug use as opposed to 8% in whites. Furthermore, black men were 20 times more likely and black women 18 times more likely than their white counterparts to have acquired HIV through IV drug use. These high figures have been attributed to the much higher prevalence of IV drug use in blacks. But it is questionable that blacks use illicit IV drugs that much more than whites. Figures on IV drug use prevalence are mostly from emergency room visits. These places tend to have an overrepresentation of blacks and thus data from such places may not give an accurate reflection of the situation.

A more likely reason is the pattern of drug use. Black IV drug users are believed to share needles more frequently. As stated in an earlier chapter, drug use itself is not as important as needle sharing in the acquisition of HIV. If, indeed, blacks share needles more frequently, then it makes sense that they would acquire HIV infection more often through IV drug use. Furthermore, black IV drug users are believed to use the most potent drugs, like "crack" cocaine; these are believed to potentiate HIV infection and progression to AIDS.

## Homosexual/Bisexual Men

Homosexual/bisexual activity accounts for the highest percentage (44%) of the distribution of AIDS by risk category in blacks. Blacks were 1.3 times more likely to acquire AIDS through homosexual activity and 3.6 times more likely through bisexual activity than whites. The reason for blacks' higher risk for AIDS through homosexual/bisexual activity has been difficult to discover. Data are not available on prevalence of homosexual/bisexual activity in blacks, but there appears to be no specific difference in black homosexual practices.

In a study of homosexuals in San Francisco, blacks were found to have a higher prevalence of HIV infection than whites; they also had a higher rate of seroconversion. The prevalence of both HIV infection and seroconversion was not explained by the number of sex partners, frequency of receptive anal/genital contact, or sharing of needles. In other words, the higher risk for blacks in this regard is unrelated to behavior. What is the reason for this excess risk? Is it due to genetic factors? Maybe—but I believe it has more to do with cofactors of infection and pathogenesis.

As discussed in Chapter 4, it has been demonstrated that individuals with certain infectious diseases such as syphilis, chancroid, hepatitis B, and herpes simplex are more likely to acquire HIV infection and progress to AIDS. Homosexuals possess these conditions more frequently than other groups. Blacks, both homosexual and heterosexual, also tend to be disproportionately represented in these conditions. A study of homosexuals in Atlanta found a decline of syphilis cases in whites between 1981 and 1985; there was an increase in blacks for the same period (Landrum et al., 1988). I suggest that the higher rate of syphilis and other (cofactor) infectious diseases in blacks is the reason for the higher risk to black homosexuals of acquiring HIV infection and AIDS.

## Heterosexual Men and Women

In the United States, 11% of AIDS cases in blacks were reported to have been acquired through heterosexual transmission as opposed to 2% in whites. Furthermore, blacks account for 61% of all cases of AIDS acquired through heterosexual transmission. Heterosexual transmission is believed to be the major means of HIV acquisition in African blacks. And heterosexual activity is believed to play a major role in HIV acquisition among Haitians.

Perhaps more than any other reason, heterosexual transmission of HIV has made the greatest contribution to speculation that blacks may be genetically more susceptible to AIDS. Eales et al. (1987) stated in their paper on the Gc gene that the fact that heterosexual spread of HIV is more common among U.S. blacks is indicative of genetic susceptibility in light of their higher frequency of Gc1F and lower frequency of Gc2. Again, I suggest that genes may play a role but the environment predominates.

I discussed in detail in Chapter 4 that access to blood is the main issue in HIV transmission irrespective of means of access. In other words, sexual activity per se is not as important as the virus' gaining access to blood. In this regard, genital lesions provide good access to the virus. And data demonstrate a higher prevalence of syphilis, chancroid, genital warts, and herpes simplex in U.S. blacks. The rate of these conditions is also very high among African blacks. In terms of progression to AIDS, the cofactor diseases discussed in this and other chapters may play a more prominent role than genes.

Finally, the high percentage of AIDS cases in U.S. blacks reported as occurring through heterosexual transmission may be questionable. It has been suggested that some black people may be reluctant to admit to IV drug use or homosexual activity and that many cases of AIDS in blacks reported as heterosexually acquired may actually have been acquired through IV drug use or homosexual activity.

## Transfusion of Blood/Blood Products

Though blood transfusion accounts for only 1% of all cases of AIDS in U.S. blacks, it has been a major risk factor for them as compared with whites. Black men were 1.2 times, black women were 1.9 times, and black children were 2.5 times more likely than their white counterparts to have acquired AIDS through blood transfusion (Selik, Castro, & Pappaioanou, 1988). Blood transfusion has been and continues to be the major means of HIV transmission in Africa, as discussed in Chapter 5. Transfusion of blood products for the treatment of hemophilia is the only risk category in which whites maintain a higher relative risk of HIV transmission than blacks. The reason for the risk of HIV acquisition through blood/blood products is rather straightforward; the more frequent the transfusion rate, the more likely the exposure to HIV-contaminated blood. In this regard, it has been suggested that hemophilia, a genetic disease, may be less common in blacks. The main question then is why blacks receive so many blood transfusions.

Anemia from all causes is a major health problem in blacks. In Africa, malaria, tuberculosis, and malnutrition often lead to low blood counts and the need for transfusion. In U.S. blacks, low birth weight appears to be major reason for the high rate of transfusion in black children. The rate of low birth weight deliveries in blacks is more than twice that of whites. Black women may receive more transfusions than white women for pregnancy-related conditions. Blacks tend to have more complicated deliveries, ectopic pregnancies, and a higher rate of birth; these often require blood transfusion.

## SOCIOECONOMIC STATUS

I stated in Chapter 1 of this book that the rate of AIDS/HIV infection is higher in U.S. blacks for the same reason the prevalence of heart disease, hypertension, stroke, diabetes, and so on is also higher. In other words, I believe genetics plays little if any role in the prevalence of AIDS in blacks. If one used prevalence rates to suggest susceptibility, then all these diseases with clearly much higher rates in blacks may be considered genetic. It is entirely possible that some of them—for example, hypertension—may have a genetic component. But I believe all those diseases and AIDS should be approached ecologically. They should be studied with the view of finding how the environment in which blacks live relates to their well-being.

The different risk groups for AIDS, as described above, in which blacks have higher rates have one thing in common—the socioeconomic environment. Socioeconomic status is usually a reflection of three achievable potentials—educational, occupational, and financial. Any or all of these contribute to the health status of individuals, families, and groups—that is, the lower the socioeconomic status, the less healthy the individual or group. As described in Chapter 2, U.S. blacks are less educated, less employed, and less rich. Many of the countries in Africa with high rates of AIDS have large population segments with little education, little employment, and little wealth. And Haiti is supposed to be the poorest country in the western hemisphere, with high rates of unemployment, illiteracy, and poverty.

It should be recognized that socioeconomic status vis-á-vis health status is a factor irrespective of race. In other words, well-educated, well-employed, and rich blacks have a higher health status than less educated, less employed, and poor whites. Among black Africans and Haitians, the relationship between socioeconomic status and health status is well demonstrated. This is the reason for the geographic distribution of AIDS/HIV infection among blacks in America. And this is also the reason for the higher rates of infection in the risk groups. Blacks have disproportionately higher rates because they are disproportionately of lower socioeconomic status.

Regarding IV drug use, the most distinguishing feature is the fact that black IV drug users tend to share needles more frequently—a reflection of low socioeconomic status. Black homosexuals' higher rates appear to be related to the frequency of syphilis, chancroid, and other STDs. A study in Atlanta on syphilis trends found that white men employed in professional and midlevel occupations had a decline in syphilis cases from 62% to 35% between 1981 and 1985. On the other hand, blacks had an increase from 18% to 75% for the same time period. Significantly, blacks were 10 times as likely as whites to be in low-income occupations and twice as likely to have less than a high school education (Landrum et al., 1988). A similar explanation— that is, higher rates of syphilis, chancroid, and other STDs—exists for the higher AIDS rates among black heterosexuals. And this phenomenon is related to low socioeconomic status. Finally, it should be obvious how socioeconomic status relates to transfusion-associated AIDS as described previously.

That socioeconomic status influences health status is nothing new or unique to certain populations or geographic areas. It has been observed for centuries that people at the lowest socioeconomic level have the highest rates of illness and death. This phenomenon has been observed throughout the world, and it is present whether dealing with infectious or noninfectious diseases. The phenomenon also exists for specific disease. For example, in the United States in 1972, individuals with incomes of less than $3,000 had three times the rate of heart disease as those with incomes of more than $15,000. Similarly, diabetes was about 3.5 times and anemia and arthritis were 2.5 times more prevalent in the poor than in the rich (Kaplan & Haan, 1987).

As stated earlier, socioeconomic status is a reflection of educational, occupational, and financial achievement. How do these factors affect health status? How do they contribute to the high illness and death rates for the poor? It appears that low income, poor nutrition, hazardous living conditions, and inadequate medical care contribute to poor health (Kaplan & Haan, 1987). These factors are more prevalent in individuals or groups of low socioeconomic status. And blacks are disproportionately represented by individuals of low socioeconomic status.

Socioeconomic status vis-á-vis health status may be explained by the Health Field concept as provided by Lalonde (1974) and Blum (1974). It states that the health status of individuals is under the influence of life-style, the environment, human biology, and the medical care system. In this regard, it has been estimated that 50% of our health is determined by life-style, 20% by environmental conditions, 20% by human biology (genetic predisposition), and 10% by the medical care system. From this breakdown, it is obvious that 80% of our health is determined by factors other than those we have at birth. Life-style, environmental conditions, and access to medical care are all related to socioeconomic status. Thus improvement in socioeconomic status appears to be more important to improving health status than genetic research and technological advancement in medical care. The World Health Organization has declared that advances in medical science have contributed less to improved health than changes in environmental conditions and favorable trends in the standard of living (WHO, 1957).

The WHO declaration has been demonstrated in many countries. As early as the nineteenth century, it was recognized that the major contributions to improved health in England and Wales were limitation in family size, increase in food supply, and healthier physical environment;

therapeutic measures contributed very little. The virtual eradication of tuberculosis from most of Great Britain and Scandinavia has been attributed to improvement in living standards, not to the use of chemotherapy. In the United States, deaths from infectious diseases such as tuberculosis, pneumonia, and influenza started a downward trend in the 1900s—well before the discovery of antibiotics—and this has been attributed to improvement in the standard of living.

The standard of living, a reflection of socioeconomic status, is a major difference between most developed nations and developing nations in terms of health status. Many developing nations have problems with population control, infectious diseases, food supply, and basic environmental quality. Medical care is targeted at saving lives instead of promoting health and preventing disease. As described above, the problems encountered in developing nations have largely been solved in developed nations through improvement in the standard of living. Their prevalence in many African countries and Haiti—that is, the low socioeconomic status of most of the populations in these countries—accounts for the low health status.

The problems encountered in developing nations are rather common in certain black communities in the United States. As described in Chapter 2, black inner-city residents have problems with high fertility rates, poor nutrition, infectious and noninfectious diseases, and overcrowded living conditions; they are involved in very few health promotion and disease prevention activities. These account for the higher rates of death from the leading causes among U.S. blacks than whites. In effect, these groups of U.S. blacks are a microcosm of those in developing countries. Thus it is clear that these U.S. blacks are less healthy because they are less educated, less employed, and less rich.

## CONCLUSION

This chapter is the most important one in this book. I have sought to shed some light on the controversy concerning blacks' suggested genetic susceptibility to AIDS/HIV infection. I have discussed various studies and views, both pro and con, regarding this issue. I have concluded that genetics plays little if any role in the pathogenesis of AIDS in blacks. I have used epidemiological and ecological principles to describe how the environment of many blacks makes them more susceptible to many different diseases. I have described why and how the socioeconomic status of blacks affects their health status in regard to these diseases. I have then concluded that the socioeconomic environment of blacks is the main contributing factor to the health status of blacks. Blacks are disproportionately of lower socioeconomic status; they have, therefore, disproportionately lower health status.

As described in Chapter 4, the transmission of HIV and the pathogenesis of AIDS are related to the person's overall health status and preexisting diseases. I have discussed in this and other chapters the overall poor health status of many black people and the high rate of diseases that promote the transmission of HIV and the pathogenesis of AIDS. All these factors are influenced by socioeconomic status. The prevalence of AIDS/HIV infection is disproportionately high in blacks because they have a disproportionately lower health status because they are of lower socioeconomic status. Therefore, to control AIDS/HIV infections—to prevent an even wider spread of HIV among U.S., African, and Haitian blacks—programs need to be developed to address blacks' overall health status. Programs need to be developed to improve their socioeconomic environment—because this is something *about which it is possible to do something.*

## REFERENCES

Blum, H. L. (1974). *Planning for health: Developmental application of social change theory.* New York: Human Science Press.

Constans, J., Viau, M., et al. (1978a). Analysis of Gc polymorphism in human populations by focusing in polyacrylamide gels: Demonstration of subtypes of the Gc1 alleles and additional Gc variants. *Human Genetics, 41,* 53-60.

Constans, J., Viau, M., et al. (1978b). Gc Subtypes demonstrated by isoelectric focussing: Further data and description of new variants among an African sample (Fula) from Senegal. *Japanese Journal of Human Genetics, 23,* 111-117.

Daiger, S. P., Brewton, G. S., et al. (1987). Genetic susceptibility to AIDS: Absence of an association with group specific component (Gc). *NEJM, 317,* 630-631.

Eales, L., Nye, K., et al. (1987). Group specific component and HIV infection. *Lancet, 1,* 1268-1269.

Eales, L. J., Parkin, J. M., et al. (1987). Association of different allelic forms of group specific component with susceptibility to and clinical manifestation of human immunodeficiency virus infection. *Lancet, 1,* 999-1002.

Enlow, R. W., Roldan, A. N., et al. (1983). Increased frequency of HLA-DR5 in lymphadenopathy stage of AIDS. *Lancet, 1,* 51.

Giles, K., Louie, L., et al. (1987). Genetic susceptibility to AIDS: Absence of an association with group specific component (Gc). *NEJM, 317*, 630-631.

Harris County Medical Society and the Houston Academy of Medicine. (1987). *AIDS: A guide for survival*. Houston, TX: Author.

Kaplan, G. A., & Haan, M. N. (1987). Socioeconomic status and health. In R. W. Analer & H. B. Dull (Eds.), *Closing the gap: The burden of unnecessary illness*. New York: Oxford University Press.

Konotey-Ahulu, F. I. D. (1972). Balanced polymorphism and hereditary qualitative and quantitative erythrocyte defects. *Ghana Medical Journal, 11*, 274-285.

Konotey-Ahulu, F. I. D. (1987). Group specific component and HIV infection. *Lancet, 1*, 1267.

Lalonde, M. (1974). *A new perspective on the health of Canadians*. Ottawa: Office of the Canadian Minister of National Health and Welfare.

Landrum, S., Beck-Sangue, C., et al. (1988). Racial trends in syphilis among men with same-sex partners in Atlanta, Georgia. *American Journal of Public Health, 78*, 66-67.

Last, J. M. (Ed.). (1983). *A dictionary of epidemiology*. New York: Oxford University Press.

Mausner, J. S., & Kramer, S. (1985). *Epidemiology: An introductory text*. Philadelphia: W. B. Saunders.

Morris, J. N. (1955). Uses of epidemiology. *British Medical Journal, 2*, 395.

Papiha, S. S. (1987). Group specific component and HIV infection. *Lancet, 1*, 1267-1268.

Scorza-Smeraldi, R. S., Fabio, G., et al. (1986). HLA-associated susceptibility to acquired immunodeficiency syndrome in Italian patients with human immunodeficiency virus infection. *Lancet, 2*, 1187-1189.

Selik, R. M., Castro, K. C., & Pappaioanou, M. (1988). Racial/ethnic differences in the risk of AIDS in the United States. *American Journal of Public Health, 78*, 1539-1545.

World Health Organization. (1957). *World Health Organization Monograph No. 34*. Geneva, Switzerland: Author.

# 7

# AIDS in Perspective

A factor whose presence can change wars, change the personality of entire populations, disturb social life, give rise to new faiths, appreciably affect music, literature, and art cannot but be the vital concern of civilized man. Disease is such a factor.

—Henry Sigerist

No disease in recent history has changed the personality of entire populations and disturbed social life the way AIDS has. With its relatively short history, AIDS has done all the things Dr. Sigerist describes and more.

Since its discovery in 1981, more has been spoken, written, and broadcast on AIDS in a relatively short period of time than any other disease in history. Almost daily, one hears on television or reads in the newspaper something about AIDS. Almost every issue of scientific journals has carried an article or articles on AIDS in recent years. Indeed, there are nearly 70 journals devoted to AIDS; and more than 10,000 articles have been written in various scientific journals. There has been an annual international conference since 1985 attracting thousands of participants from all over the world during which high-powered scientific research has been presented and discussed. There have been hundreds of regional and local conferences with similar presentations and discussions throughout the world.

In the United States, there has been an explosion of organizations, agencies, and foundations devoted to AIDS activity. Hundreds of special interest groups have been formed to deal with various aspects of AIDS. Many policy documents have been formulated; laws have been

passed by the U.S. Congress and state legislatures; and the courts
have issued various pronouncements. Businesses, governmental agencies, schools, hospitals, and prisons have developed workplace policies
on AIDS. There have been thousands of symposia and in-service programs in schools, hospitals, and other work sites on AIDS.

All the conferences, policies, and legislation aim to educate the
public. With such a massive information explosion, one would expect
a reasonably informed public, at least in the United States, as far as
knowledge about AIDS is concerned. But there also is widespread
hysteria and apprehension concerning AIDS. "Horror" stories abound;
and many incidents demonstrate widespread ignorance about the disease.

I have been giving speeches on AIDS for several years. I have spoken to doctors, other hospital and health care employees, news media
personnel, and the general public. I have been invited by businesses,
hospital boards, and school boards to help develop workplace policies
on AIDS. During these presentations, I have heard questions and
comments that demonstrate profound ignorance. In most of my presentations, I start by telling stories that display ignorance and empha-
size the need to know more about the disease. The following are some
of the stories.

A young man with AIDS living in Houston went to his hometown,
a small town in Texas, to die as his disease progressed. His parents
did not know he had AIDS; neither did they know he was homosexual. When his condition deteriorated to near death, he complained of
chest pain and was put in a local hospital. During a visit by his
mother, a nurse happened to mention that the patient had AIDS. The
mother ran to the bathroom, vomited, and came back to the patient's
bedside to say, "I'll never see you again as long as you live." She did
not return to the hospital until the son died a few days later.

A young man in his late thirties worked for the Houston school district. As part of his job, he and a coworker visited the home of a
school district employee to discuss some business matters. On their
way back to the office, his friend mentioned that the employee they
visited had AIDS. The young man became upset that the authorities
had not informed him of that person's having AIDS. On arrival at his
home, he stood in the doorway and took off his clothes. He had sat on
the AIDS victim's couch, and he thought that if he did not take off his
clothes before sitting on his own couch, he would give AIDS to his
wife and young children.

During the national AIDS conference in San Francisco in November 1987, the following story was told by an attorney to the conferees: A woman went to her boss to ask for permission to take some time off to spend time with her husband who was in the hospital with AIDS. Without responding directly to the woman's request, the boss gave her an ultimatum: get a blood test for AIDS once a month and provide him with the results or be terminated from the job. The woman consulted the attorney, and, when the attorney contacted the employer, his response was that he had a responsibility to protect other employees from catching AIDS from the woman—"she uses [the same] telephones, water fountains, and toilets as other employees," he concluded.

The above stories illustrate the apprehension many people still have about AIDS, despite the glut of information about the disease. This level of apprehension exists despite the information explosion because many people, throughout the entire population, do not understand the disease. More stories follow.

In a small town in Texas, it became known to the manager of a fast-food restaurant that one of his employees had tested positive for HIV antibodies. This employee was a janitor who did not handle food. Because of fear of the employee's passing on the virus to other employees and customers, the manager was faced with the dilemma of dismissing or keeping the employee. He approached the local family physician for advice. The doctor decided to evaluate the employee before making a recommendation. The employee waited in the doctor's waiting room at the appointed time. When the doctor came out of his office to get the employee, he opened the door half way, stuck his head out to call the patient, and had a face mask covering his mouth and nose.

Even a doctor can believe that, if an HIV-antibody-positive person breathes on him, he could acquire the virus. This incident occurred in 1987, six years after the discovery of AIDS and despite thousands of articles on the subject.

There are many more stories like those narrated above throughout the United States. AIDS victims have lost their jobs, houses/apartments, and insurance policies. Some doctors have refused to take care of AIDS patients. Some doctors, particularly surgeons, have sought to test certain patients or all patients for HIV antibodies before performing certain procedures. Worse is that certain patients are tested without their knowledge. I know of at least one case in a major university medical center in Texas where a patient was tested without his knowledge. The patient had been admitted for elective surgery. Blood was drawn for routine preoperative tests, and some of the blood was used for an HIV-antibody test. When the test came back positive, the patient was discharged without surgery and without being told why he had been discharged.

Why is there such apprehension about AIDS, despite the fact that so much has been written and said about it? I have observed that, regarding AIDS education, the public is given *facts* instead of *understandable and useful information*. Lack of understanding, I believe, is the reason for the hysteria about AIDS. While the public may not have understandable and useful information, some doctors also simply have not taken the time to understand AIDS. Thousands of scientific papers are available for doctors to read and understand; hundreds of conferences and symposia have been held. But many doctors have not taken advantage of these papers and conferences to educate themselves and then to educate the public. I conducted a survey on AIDS in which simple questions—but ones that required a fairly good understanding of AIDS for correct answers—were asked. Doctors and other health care workers scored as low as members of the public.

AIDS is a new disease that has spread rather fast throughout the world. Because of its communicability and fatality, and, perhaps more important, because of the segments of population it affected initially (homosexuals and IV drug users), people have reacted to the disease with their "hearts" instead of their "heads." By *heart* and *head* I mean that people have reacted to AIDS emotionally instead of thoughtfully and analytically. For an epidemic disease with complex biochemical and psychosocial parameters, facts alone are not likely to effect a transfer of reaction from the heart to the head. Educational messages to the public should be understandable and persuasive; simply disseminating facts is not likely to persuade the public.

I believe failure to effectively educate the public has led to widespread apprehension about AIDS, as evidenced by the stories narrated above. Other stories of school and work boycotts because of the presence of individuals with AIDS or who are HIV-antibody positive have been publicized. The Ryan White story is well known. This boy was 12 years old when diagnosed with AIDS as a result of frequent blood factor transfusions for hemophilia. His school was boycotted; he was ridiculed by schoolmates and neighbors; and people shot at his house. The family finally moved from their hometown of Kokomo, Indiana.

In Arcadia, Florida, two boys in the Ray family had hemophilia. The boys tested positive for HIV antibodies, and somehow word got around the town that the children had AIDS. People started shunning the family, and the parents approached the minister of their church for support. Upon hearing the HIV status of the boys, the minister recommended to the church session that the family be kicked out and be barred from attending church. This led to an uproar in the town, with demands that the boys be barred from school, indeed, be expelled from the town. The family's house was burned down, and they finally moved from Arcadia.

Both news reports and protestors in Arcadia kept referring to the children as having AIDS—a gross misunderstanding of the disease process. Confusing HIV-antibody positivity with AIDS is rather common among many people, including some health professionals (as seen in the survey referred to earlier). This and many other aspects of the AIDS issue are misunderstood because people do not view it in perspective.

## AIDS IN PERSPECTIVE

In most of my presentations on AIDS, I write on a chalkboard or show a slide of the outline of my speech; the last item in the outline is "AIDS in Perspective." This is the time during the presentation when I try to engage the audience more actively, try to get them to think of what I had discussed up to that point. I had discussed epidemiology, transmission and pathogenesis, and clinical manifestations and treatment. At this point, I pose rhetorical questions to stimulate thinking and discussion. I call attention to certain issues in such a manner as might not have occurred to them before—all with the idea that we need to approach AIDS thoughtfully instead of emotionally.

People have approached AIDS emotionally by and large because of the perception that the two main means of transmission (homosexuality and IV drug use) involve immoral and criminal activity. In effect, AIDS victims brought their plight upon themselves. Why should the rest of us worry about them? When they are going to die anyway, why should society spend time and money on them? I heard a prominent Texas politician in 1987 make this remark: "If these bastards [referring to homosexuals and IV drug users] did not indulge in their disgusting behavior, we won't have this problem [AIDS]."

Even those of us who do not fall into the politician's categories have our own "disgusting" behaviors. We know that cigarette smoking is bad for us—it kills thousands of people and costs billions of dollars—yet we smoke. We know that too much alcohol and too much food cause disease, yet we eat and drink excessively. We know drinking and driving cause death and injury, yet we drink and drive. We know seat belts save lives, yet we drive without wearing seat belts.

Politicians and health officials alike lament the financial cost of AIDS and make statements that imply blame for the victims. They often quote figures, such as that AIDS will cost the United States $16 billion dollars by 1991. Let us look at that figure in perspective. AIDS may cost the nation $16 billion in 10 years; cigarette smoking costs $65 billion *per year*. AIDS is expected to kill about 170,000 Americans by 1991—in 10 years—cigarette smoking kills 390,000 Americans *per year*. Keep in mind that cigarette smokers have deliberately chosen a life-style, a behavior, that causes hundreds of thousands of deaths and costs billions of dollars annually. How much different are cigarette smokers than homosexuals and IV drug users? Cigarette smoking kills more people in the United States than illicit drug use, alcohol, AIDS, and accidents combined.

I had heard and read about scientists lamenting the shortage of research dollars: There is a shortage of research money because funds that could otherwise add to those for cancer, heart disease, and other diseases are being used for AIDS. Again, some of these people make statements that tend to blame AIDS victims. The most pervasive and appalling of such statements I have heard was made by Dr. Marshall Goldberg on NBC's *Today Show*.

On August 21, 1988, Dr. Goldberg was being interviewed on the *Today Show* on his newly published book on the use of monoclonal antibodies to treat cancer. He called for more research in this area toward more effective treatment and the possible cure of cancer. He regretted that AIDS is taking research money away from other research activities; because of AIDS there is a shortage of both money and personnel for cancer research "and cancer happens to nicer people," he concluded.

It is estimated that cigarette smoking is responsible for 33% of all cancers, and diet accounts for nearly 40% of cancers. It can be said then that cancer victims chose to smoke cigarettes or eat too much of the wrong things; they brought their disease upon themselves. How much "nicer" are cancer victims than AIDS victims?

I suppose it is not surprising to hear lay people make prejudicial statements about AIDS victims if physicians like Dr. Goldberg can make such a statement. On another television show, a family physician in Phoenix, Arizona, who took care of most of the AIDS patients in that city, related that some doctors who saw his patients during his absence had told some of the patients (mostly homosexuals) that they deserved the disease. On a television talk show, one guest was a homosexual with AIDS. A member of the audience got up and literally shouted: "I'm repulsed by the man's life-style; I'm repulsed by his disease; and I'm repulsed by him," and the audience applauded.

The discussion in the last several paragraphs reflects my concern about the view that AIDS is somehow a disease of unclean and immoral people or criminals. There is no way of knowing whether AIDS would have occurred had there been no homosexual activity or IV drug use. Suppose it were truly the case—that is, that there would be no AIDS if not for homosexual activity and IV drug use. AIDS is here, and society must deal with it. The same type of prejudicial attitude is not directed toward victims of other diseases equally involving life-style and personal choices; why should AIDS be different? And, more important, if the AIDS epidemic is not halted, it will eventually affect every segment of society.

## Legal Means of Control

Because people often perceive of AIDS in moral and criminal terms, attempts have been made to control the epidemic through legal instead of public health means. Proposed and enacted legislation abounds at federal, state, and local levels. There is legislation on isolation and quarantine, reporting, screening, education (what can be taught in schools), and prosecution of individuals who transmit HIV to others. One of the most publicized and controversial is legislation on premarital screening. It has been proposed in many states; and the state of Illinois has made HIV-antibody testing a requirement for a marriage license. Figures from that state show that only 5 out of 44,726 tests have been positive. The Illinois legislature is considering a repeal of the law (Gostlin, 1989).

Requiring HIV-antibody testing for a marriage license is both too costly and ineffective in terms of prevention of HIV transmission. Gostlin quotes costs of finding one HIV-antibody-positive individual through premarital screening as being between $60,000 and $100,000;

so this type of screening is obviously not worth the cost. In addition, even if a reasonable number of cases were identified, this type of screening is not likely to accomplish the goal of preventing HIV transmission; most couples seeking marriage licenses have already had sexual contact. Indeed, those likely to test positive are more likely to engage in premarital sex.

Many proponents of HIV premarital screening use syphilis premarital screening to justify their position. I heard Sam Donaldson say on ABC's *This Week with David Brinkley* that when he was growing up, blood tests for syphilis were required for marriage licenses. He saw no reason the same should not be required for HIV. What he did not know, or failed to consider, was the reasoning behind the proposal to require syphilis testing for marriage licenses. With the effective use of penicillin to cure syphilis, the plan was to eradicate syphilis through case identification. Screening through premarital blood testing would identify cases who could be brought to treatment. The eradication program did not succeed, and most states stopped requiring syphilis testing for marriage licenses in the 1980s.

There is no cure or effective treatment for HIV; therefore, mass screening for eradication purposes would be ineffective. What did the legislators of Illinois plan to do with HIV test results other than notifying the couple? The implication is that a couple receiving a positive test result would cancel their marriage plans, despite the fact that the Illinois law allows subsequent granting of a marriage license. Studies have shown that most couples would proceed with marriage plans after receiving positive HIV test results. So the use of a program like the one attempted for syphilis eradication to justify premarital HIV testing implies a shortsighted approach to a complex problem.

Another legal approach to the AIDS epidemic is making the transmission of HIV a criminal offense. Many states have statutes making it a criminal offense for a person with HIV infection to knowingly engage in needle sharing or sexual intercourse without informing the partner. Individuals accused of the above offenses, plus such trivial ones as spitting, biting, and splashing of blood, have been prosecuted. Some of these offenses carry rather stiff penalties; for example, Louisiana and South Carolina have maximum sentences of $5,000 and 10 years' imprisonment (Gostlin, 1989).

To be sure, many states also have statues on confidentiality regarding HIV testing and discrimination against AIDS/HIV-infected patients.

Laudable as these statutes are, the many more statutes on the issues discussed above appear to discriminate against AIDS victims. No other disease, even those that kill more people and cost society more money, has so many regulations and potential penalties. Furthermore, the legal approach tends to hinder public health efforts in the control of the epidemic. As is well known, education is the best—indeed, the only—weapon currently available to curb the spread of HIV. One of the public health approaches to education is testing and counseling. If coercion and threat of prosecution are used to get people tested, many would not come forward to be tested. People who may be engaging in high-risk behavior and should be targeted for testing and counseling may not be reached.

### Discrimation and Victim Stereotyping

As stated earlier, I believe the reaction of individuals and institutions to AIDS—that is, more often emotional instead of thoughtful—is influenced by the perception that AIDS is a disease of "undesirables." A Dallas county commissioner made a comment on television some time ago during an interview about the fact that Dallas County (with the second largest number of AIDS cases in Texas) was spending so little money on AIDS. His response was that there was no money. The interviewer asked whether the county commission would consider raising money for AIDS through taxes. The commissioner's response: "Taxpayers won't go for it . . . they might be willing to pay taxes for *terminal* cancer or *terminal* [italics added] heart disease but not AIDS."

It is often argued that AIDS patients are going to die anyway, so why spend money on them. This commissioner above seems to believe that it is OK to spend money on *terminal* cancer and heart disease patients. Are they not going to die anyway? The statement displays a clear inconsistency—indeed, a discriminatory attitude—vis-á-vis AIDS victims that seems rather widespread. Heart disease and cancer are mostly the result of life-style; cigarette smoking, dietary indiscretion, and lack of exercise account for the majority of heart disease and cancer. Yet nobody attempts to deny victims of these diseases access to treatment. Millions of dollars are spent annually in the United States on research and therapy on these two killer diseases. The cost of AIDS in terms of lives and money does not even come close to that for heart disease and cancer. I wondered how the man who made the comment above, who was quite obese, would react if he was brought to my emergency room with a heart attack (with the potential of death) and I told him he would not be treated because he got his heart disease from eating too much fatty food and not exercising.

The sentiment expressed by the county commissioner seems to be the view of many physicians and other health care workers. Often, health care workers express unwillingness to deal with AIDS patients ostensibly from fear of acquiring HIV. I believe it is more from fear of acquiring AIDS. Some people would rather be shot to death than get AIDS lest they be identified with the "undesirables" of society. I hold this view based on comments I have heard over the years. Furthermore, these health care workers do not hesitate to treat patients with other communicable diseases, some as deadly as AIDS. For example, hepatitis acquired from patients kills about 250 health care workers each year in the United States. Not a single death from AIDS has occurred so far through workplace acquisition.

Many times, when scientific data are cited in an attempt to calm fears about AIDS, it is countered that AIDS is a new disease; we don't know enough about it, so we should not take chances. It is true that AIDS is a new disease and knowledge about it is evolving, but enough information exists so that AIDS patients can be cared for with appropriate precautions. In addition, people do not seem to question available scientific data on other diseases. Two recently discovered diseases—Legionnaires' disease and Lyme disease—are examples. They, like AIDS, seem to have come from nowhere. When their existence became known, scientists went to work to aggressively pursue the cause. The causative agents were discovered; treatment protocols were developed; and control measures were established. Health professionals and the public accepted what researchers said about the diseases, and there was no an outcry about not knowing enough about them.

Legionnaires' disease was unknown prior to 1976. In the summer of 1976, a group of American Legion members were having their annual meeting at the Bellevue Stratford Hotel in Philadelphia when some of them suddenly became ill. They had similar symptoms—high fever, shaking chills, cough, chest pain, and diarrhea. Epidemiologists from the CDC and other scientists started an aggressive investigation that led to implication of watercoolers in the hotel's air-conditioning system. A new bacterium was isolated as the causative agent of the illness, and it was named *Legionella pneumophila*. Since the Philadelphia outbreak, several outbreaks have occurred, usually associated with buildings such as hospitals and hotels. *Legionella pneumophila* has been isolated from other water sources such as lakes, creeks, ponds, and hot water tanks. It is believed to be transmitted by the airborne route. There is no evidence that person-to-person transmission occurs.

Lyme disease was unknown prior to 1975. In that year, the Connecticut State Department of Health received calls on unusually large numbers of arthritis cases occurring in the town of Lyme, Connecticut. Scientists, especially Dr. Allen Steare, started to investigate, and the investigation led to some common symptomatology in most of the patients: The onset of the illness was mostly in the summer and early fall; a peculiar rash often preceded the arthritic symptoms; and many of the patients recalled a tick bite at the site of the rash. Further investigation led to identification of a new tick species that was named *Ixodes dammini.* In 1981, a bacterium (a spirochete) was isolated from *Ixodes dammini,* and blood from some patients suffering from the symptoms described above tested positive for antibodies to the spirochete. The spirochete has been named *Borrelia burgborferi.*

Since the epidemic in Connecticut, many cases have been identified in most states in the United States and several other countries. Further research has led to the discovery of other symptoms involving the heart and the central nervous system. The spirochete is believed to be transmitted through tick bite only. There is no evidence of person-to-person transmission.

The two newly discovered diseases discussed above have several things in common with AIDS. All three seem to have sprung from nowhere; they all started in a group or specific area in epidemic proportions and were later identified in many populations and geographic areas; they all involve a previously unknown microorganism. Perhaps most significant is the vigor and speed with which scientific investigation proceeded to discover the causative agents of the three diseases. And most intriguing is the fact that these "newly discovered" diseases may all have existed long before their "discovery." Legionnaires' disease has been traced back to 1947, with an outbreak in the United States in 1965; the characteristic skin rash of Lyme disease called *erythema chronicum migrans* was described by Swedish scientists in 1909 to have occurred after a tick bite; and HIV has been isolated from blood stored since the 1950s in different geographic regions.

As stated earlier, there has not been an outcry about what is really known about Legionnaires' disease and Lyme disease. But people, including many health professionals, continue to question data on AIDS. People ask whether it can be stated for sure that HIV is not transmitted through food, handshake, or mosquito bite. Indeed, I have been asked whether I could prove that the transmission of HIV does not occur by those processes. It is not enough, I am told, to say this is the case as far as we know or as current data show. We need proof. To insist on such proof is counter to the nature of scientific process. Scientific information and knowledge are acquired based on the *best available* data, not absolute proof. No disease has been absolutely proved to occur in certain ways. Through epidemiological, basic science, and clinical science investigation, certain conclusions are reached about the characteristics of diseases. Based on such conclusions, therapeutic and other control measures are devised that are accepted as standards.

Such is the approach to scientific research and disease investigation. This is tradition; and it is seldom, if ever, questioned. There is no way to absolutely prove cause and effect. For example, nobody knows for sure that *Legionella pneumophila* causes Legionnaires' disease or *Borrelia burgborferi* causes Lyme disease. Also, nobody knows for sure that Legionnaires' disease and Lyme disease are not transmitted from person to person. Yet such parameters have been accepted. Why then do people have difficulty accepting what is known about AIDS? Again, I believe this has to do with the fact that AIDS has been associated with the undesirables of society, and some people want to avoid it all costs. It is OK to avoid any disease, especially a fatal one, but we should not go overboard, that is, to the point of overt discrimination, in our attempt to avoid AIDS.

I have often discussed cigarette smoking at length in my presentations on AIDS. I wonder why society accepts smoking but condemns IV drug use and homosexual activity. Smoking is a personal choice; it causes disease and death; and it costs society billions of dollars, just as IV drug use and homosexual activity are personal choices and may involve disease and death. More important, the cost of cigarette smoking in terms of life and money is much higher than that of IV drug use and homosexual activity.

I posed this question—why society accepts cigarette smoking?—during a presentation on AIDS some time ago, and a member of the audience responded that cigarette smoking is not a communicable disease as is AIDS. My response was that *it is communicable*. Second-hand smoking is known to cause or exacerbate respiratory diseases in family members and coworkers of smokers. Adenocarcinoma of the lung and cervical cancer are known to be associated with secondhand smoking. Furthermore, smoking is communicable in that pregnant smokers pass disease on to their fetuses resulting in miscarriages, low birth weight deliveries, and increased neonatal mortality. So the argument that smoking is purely a personal choice—that it is OK to smoke because smokers harm themselves and nobody else—is invalid. Smokers harm others through secondhand smoking and harm society through increased health care and other costs.

Cigarette smoking is the single most preventable cause of illness and premature death in the United States. Smokers have a more than 70% greater rate of death from all causes than nonsmokers. Smoking is responsible for more than 390,000 deaths annually, which is more than 1,000 deaths *daily*; and over 10 million people suffer from chronic diseases associated with cigarette smoking in the United States alone.

Cigarette smoking is associated with the following cancers: cancer of the lung, larynx, pharynx, mouth, throat, pancreas, cervix, and bladder. It is associated with angina, heart attack, atherosclerosis, bronchitis, emphysema, peptic ulcer, and leg claudication. More significant is the effect of smoking on nonsmokers. Pregnant smokers have more miscarriages, low birth weight infants, and higher neonatal death rates. Family members, especially children, of smokers experience more respiratory infections. And secondhand smoking by family members and coworkers exacerbates such conditions as sinusitis, hay fever, and asthma. Finally, cigarette smoking costs U.S. citizens more than $65 billion annually through health care, fires, lost productivity, insurance, and compensation claims.

These are some of the health and economic costs of cigarette smoking to individuals and society. But, as individuals and as a society, we seem to have accepted smoking as part of life. On the other hand, we react emotionally to so-called killer diseases, AIDS being an example. Despite scientific evidence that HIV requires some direct contact for transmission, many people would not want to work in the same office or live near AIDS patients. Yet, despite scientific evidence on effects of secondhand smoking, we allow people to smoke in enclosed offices, airplanes, and even hospitals. And some parents who would not allow their children to attend school with an AIDS victim would not hesitate to smoke in a room or car with those children.

As stated earlier, the cost of cigarette smoking to society is much higher than the cost of AIDS. It is interesting that some of the loudest "protestors" against AIDS promote smoking; Senator Jesse Helms of North Carolina is such a person. He proposed a bill to require all food handlers to be tested for HIV antibodies (believing, I suppose, that HIV is transmitted through food). The so-called Helms amendment, attached to President Reagan's 1989 AIDS budget, prohibited federal funding to any agency for AIDS that teaches or promotes homosexuality. Senator Helms demonstrated a lack of understanding of AIDS in wanting to test food handlers. He also implies that AIDS is a homosexual disease. On the other hand, he is a strong advocate for smoking. He has vehemently opposed propositions to increase taxes on cigarettes and a ban on cigarette advertising. He even wrote a letter to the Japanese prime minister complaining about barriers to U.S. tobacco imports to Japan.

The same hypocrisy also is demonstrated by the U.S. government. As part of its so-called war on drugs, the U.S. government has threatened trade sanctions against many foreign governments from whose countries cocaine and other illicit drugs come to United States. President Reagan even deployed the U.S. Army in Bolivia to help curb cocaine production. On the other hand, foreign governments are threatened with trade sanctions for having barriers to U.S. tobacco product imports. A special effort has been made by the U.S. government and U.S. tobacco companies to increase cigarette consumption in Asia; countries like Taiwan, the Philippines, and Thailand have been targeted. The U.S. State Department has ordered all U.S. ambassadors to exert pressure on Asian governments to allow or increase the importation of U.S. cigarettes or suffer the consequence of sanctions on Asian textile and other products (Wilde, 1989).

When nonsmokers complain about smoking in public, smokers (and some nonsmokers) counter that they have a right to smoke wherever they choose, forgetting that nonsmokers have the right to breathe clean air. During my third year of medical school, I took a pack of cigarettes away from a patient, and the resident who supervised me got upset. I had convinced one of the patients who had been assigned to me not to smoke while in the hospital. I convinced him that smoking was interfering with the healing process; in addition, it was dangerous to smoke in bed (he was too sick to even sit up, let alone get out of bed). He stated that he would not smoke, and I asked him to give the cigarettes to me lest he be tempted to smoke. Unfortunately, the resident feared infringing upon the patient's civil rights and warned me not to go to such a drastic extent in my patient education efforts.

Yes, many doctors and other health professionals believe that smokers have the right to smoke, although the health consequences of smoking are well known. Therefore, patients with angina, heart attack, pneumonia, emphysema, asthma, and peptic ulcer are allowed to smoke in the hospital. Treatment is not denied (and should not be denied) patients with smoking-induced diseases even when it is clear that they are going to die. Yet, as stated earlier, treatment has been denied AIDS patients purportedly because they are going to die. Even worse is the denial of treatment to patients positive for HIV antibodies with no evidence of AIDS. I have always believed that refusal to care for AIDS/HIV-infected patients has little to do with the fact that they are going to die; it has more to do with health professionals' fear of contracting HIV.

A family physician in California had a patient with pneumonia and endocarditis. An infectious disease specialist was consulted. The patient had a history of drug abuse and had had two HIV-antibody tests, the first positive and the second negative, three years earlier. She had no opportunistic infections or other symptoms of AIDS. Yet, the infectious disease specialist wrote on the patient's chart that she had AIDS and recommended that she have surgery for the endocarditis. The surgeon refused to do surgery, and the reason both specialists gave was that the patient had a low probability of surviving for five years. When the surgeon was pressed by the family physician, he responded that he did not want to put the operating room personnel and himself at risk. Then the family physician asked what the surgeon would do if the patient had been a vice president of a local bank who acquired HIV through blood transfusion. The surgeon's reply: "To be honest, I'd operate." He added that the patient's life-style made long-term survival less likely. He refused to operate, and the patient died several days later (Wake, 1989).

The story demonstrates how society treats its poor citizens. The patient had been seen by the doctor in his office on a Friday with fever, cough, shortness of breath, and body aches. She did not have insurance, so the doctor forwent the chest X-ray and blood test he had wanted to confirm the diagnosis of pneumonia. He gave her an antibiotic and sent her home. Her condition deteriorated during the weekend, and she ended up in an intensive care unit where she died because the surgeon would not operate on her. If the X-ray and blood tests had been done, the patient might have been admitted to the hospital on Friday, where a more effective therapy would have been instituted. And if the patient had not been poor, she would have had the operation. The article in which this story appeared was titled: "How Many Patients Will Die Because We Fear AIDS."

Lack of access to health care for the poor has been a long-standing problem in U.S. society, and it has become more glaring since the AIDS epidemic. Because of discrimination against AIDS patients, mainly those who acquired the disease through homosexual activity and IV drug use, many of them have lost their jobs and insurance. They have had to depend upon public assistance, which means being seen in substandard clinics and being admitted to public hospitals. In these places, they often encounter health care workers who are reluctant to take care of them. When workers are willing to proceed, there is sometimes a shortage of resources or facilities, and these patients may not undergo needed diagnostic procedures or therapy.

When the poor are very sick and are likely to die, we tend to question the need to use all available resources to keep them alive. This is particularly true when the illnesses could be blamed on them. However, when the well-to-do are in a similar situation, we spare no expense to keep them alive even when it is clear they will ultimately die and the illnesses could be "blamed" on them. I have seen patients with terminal lung cancer (acquired from years of smoking) undergo expensive diagnostic and therapeutic procedures. We are often told by family members to do everything possible to keep such patients alive, and we comply to the extent of putting them on respirators. Is it OK to do as much as possible for lung cancer patients who acquired their disease through a personal choice but not OK to do the same for AIDS patients? Is it OK to "go all the way" with terminal lung cancer patients when we know they are going to die but not do the same for AIDS patients?

I have attempted here to shed a little more light on the inconsistency of our approach to "conventional" medical problems vis-à-vis AIDS. The inconsistency sometimes borders on discrimination. The discriminatory attitude appears to stem from the fear of AIDS, not so much as a deadly disease but as a disease of the underclass, of undesirables. Also, the fear stems from lack of understanding of AIDS as a disease entity.

As discussed in the last chapter, disease has a lot to do with the state of being of the individual before exposure to a causative agent.

Therefore, whether one acquires a disease depends upon one's health status—genetic, environmental, and socioeconomic. Socioeconomic status seems to be the predominant determinant of health and, consequently, of disease. Black people have had relatively low socioeconomic status. This has led to low health status and higher rates of most diseases. It is not surprising that they should have disproportionately high rates of AIDS. It should be emphasized again that the high numbers of black AIDS cases are predominantly among poor, inner-city blacks, not all blacks; that is, AIDS in blacks is not a genetic disease.

The discriminatory attitude toward AIDS patients seems to be related to the fact that the disease was first seen among homosexuals and IV drug users; and homosexual activity and IV drug use are viewed by many as immoral or criminal. There should be no justification for such discrimination because we do not discriminate against people with diseases caused by cigarette smoking, for example. As more cases of AIDS occur in blacks, the discrimination against homosexuals and IV drug users could spread to blacks. It is more dangerous because it is much easier to identify a person by color than by homosexual activity or IV drug use. Discrimination against black AIDS patients puts them in a vicious circle. Their health status, which often puts them at a greater risk of acquiring AIDS, resulted from their having a high rate of poverty. The high poverty rate is related to a long history of discrimination in education and employment. So discrimination in education and employment has led to poverty, which has led to poor health status, which has led to high rates of many diseases including AIDS.

Discrimination against black AIDS patients (as against all AIDS patients) is not as serious as labeling AIDS a disease of blacks. What is likely to happen is that black people, particularly poor inner-city blacks, will all be suspects when seeking medical care. Health care providers may be more reluctant to care for blacks until they are sure of their HIV-antibody status. And more blacks are likely to be tested without their knowledge for HIV antibodies.

Another type of discrimination against blacks is through international travel. This has already started, as several countries require HIV-antibody testing for entry. Belgium, for example, requires African nationals to test negative for HIV antibodies before entering the country; it does not require Belgian nationals to be tested before going to Africa. The United States requires HIV-antibody testing for all immigrant applicants. Though this is universal, it has the potential for discrimination against African applicants because of the relatively high false positive rates among Africans. Many African countries do not have enough or proper testing equipment; and other diseases such as malaria may give a false positive HIV-antibody result. This will effectively keep many Africans from immigrating to the United States.

Perhaps the best (or the worst) example of discrimination against black people in terms of AIDS is the incident at Nanking University in China. In December 1988, African students at the university were harassed by Chinese students because of fear of AIDS in the African students. The Africans protested, and some of them requested to be returned home. The university authorities, in an attempt to solve the problem, asked for decreased social contact between African and Chinese students. The remarkable thing about this incident is that the official position reinforced the Chinese students' fears; that is, the authorities asked for decreased contact between the two student groups to prevent transmission of HIV from the Africans. Being born in an African country should not make a student suspect for HIV infection. This is equivalent to other racial stereotyping that has been denounced by progressive people all over the world.

As we protest racial discrimination in South Africa; as we protest human rights abuses in such countries as the Soviet Union, Cuba, and Chile; as we protest the killing of Palestinians by Israeli soldiers, we should be mindful of the potential and real discrimination against all AIDS patients and black AIDS patients in particular.

U.S. blacks have mostly been in the underclass of U.S. society since their arrival in the New World. They started living as slaves, and slavery is the lowest form of human suppression and discrimination. With the abolition of slavery, many of them were able to undertake various endeavors to better themselves. Real advancement started in the 1950s with the inception of the civil rights movement, culminating with the passing of several civil rights laws during the Johnson administration in the 1960s. These laws eliminated virtually all forms of legal discrimination. For the first time, blacks had the chance to compete with the rest of Americans for educational and employment opportunities. But the competition was not on a level field. It is tantamount to two people's running a 100-meter dash race. One stands at the zero line, the other stands at the 20-meter line; but the whistle goes for them to start at the same time. Unless the one at the zero line is superhuman, there is no way for him to catch up with the one at the 20-meter line. So, starting from behind, most blacks have been unable to catch up with whites in terms of economic success.

Affirmative action laws gave some advantages to some blacks for educational and employment opportunities but the majority of them have been struggling. The civil rights gains by blacks in the 1960s have, by and large, given way to so-called institutional racism in the 1970s and 1980s. The civil rights gains in the 1960s were mostly in the form of political freedom; in the 1970s and 1980s, blacks found themselves mostly without economic freedom. They are usually less educated; they usually take the most menial and lowest-paying jobs; they usually live in less than adequate housing; they usually have the highest rates of unemployment and poverty—and they usually have the highest prevalence rates for most diseases.

It should be emphasized that many blacks have achieved the "American Dream." It is poor blacks who mostly suffer from institutional racism, who seem to have little chance to achieve any degree of personal advancement. It is poor blacks who have the highest rates of diseases. And it is mostly poor blacks who continue to experience various forms of discrimination, including that for AIDS. In essence, discrimination affects them more as poor people than as blacks. The "war on drugs" illustrates this point.

When politicians talk about the "drug epidemic," they usually refer to inner-city residents of housing projects who deal in "crack." The war on drugs is often directed at those residents within a large population of poor blacks. Police raids at such housing projects with arrests and jailings are not uncommon. On the other hand, politicians, movie and television actors/actresses, musicians, and athletes who indulge in illicit drug use are treated very gently. These famous and usually very rich individuals are sent off to some "paradise" drug treatment center for treatment. In March 1989, I heard Senator Phil Gramm of Texas announce on TV that the U.S. Congress would soon pass a law to throw out residents of government housing who were caught dealing in drugs. But the harshest penalty for the famous people indulging in the same activity usually is a fine, which they easily pay. Significantly, these famous people include blacks. Dwight Gooden and Lawrence Taylor, two millionaire black athletes, are examples of famous people who have been given "royal" treatment after being caught for using cocaine.

The idea that illicit drug use is mainly (or only, in some people's minds) the problem of poor blacks is often graphically displayed by the news media. On April 4, 1989, the NBC television program *The*

*Today Show* was devoted entirely to the drug problem in the United States. The opening segment showed a police raid of a housing project inhabited by poor blacks. A long segment was on scientific research dealing with the effect of cocaine on the human brain. People indulging in cocaine were shown; some were in homes or apartments, others were at drug treatment centers. Several of the drug users were interviewed; every one of the drug users shown was black and poor.

In March 1989, in the city of Waco, Texas, police organized a series of weekend raids on illicit drug users. The television cameras accompanied the police, and the raids were graphically shown during the news broadcasts. The raids were only at housing projects. On March 23, 1989, the leading story of one of the local television evening news reports was a raid on a housing project inhabited by poor blacks. People were shown being wrestled down by police and handcuffed. Some of the men were not wearing shirts. The reporter discussed how easy it was to purchase drugs in the project and that even children were involved in drug dealing. The conclusion was that the whole project was infested with illicit drugs. This story was immediately followed by another drug story. This one involved a white man who was being tried for possessing millions of dollars worth of cocaine. A different reporter discussed in some detail the background of the accused—his hometown, family status, the college he had attended and his major field of study as well as his workplace. Furthermore, every time the camera was focused on the accused, his face was deliberately distorted to protect his identity.

At this particular television station, there are glaring differences in the reporting of criminal activities involving illicit drugs. Poor blacks were shown being dragged from their apartments without the benefit, in some cases, of adequate clothing. They were depicted as hopeless and irresponsible people. On the other hand, the white man was not photographed during the arrest. He was shown in a courtroom wearing a nice suit, and the pictures of his face were distorted. He was depicted as a responsible citizen who had somehow gone (or been led) astray.

## CONCLUSION

I maintain that there would not be such a high level of fear of AIDS, and thus potential and real discrimination against AIDS

**Table 7.1**   The 15 Leading Causes of Death per 100,000 Population:
United States, 1987

| Cause of Death | | Rate | Percentage of Total |
|---|---|---|---|
| All causes | | 872.4 | 100.0 |
| 1. | Diseases of the heart | 312.4 | 35.8 |
| 2. | Malignant neoplasm | 195.9 | 22.5 |
| 3. | Cerebrovascular disease | 61.6 | 7.1 |
| 4. | Accidents and adverse effects | 39.0 | 4.5 |
| 5. | Chronic obstructive pulmonary diseases | 32.2 | 3.7 |
| 6. | Pneumonia and influenza | 28.4 | 3.3 |
| 7. | Diabetes mellitus | 15.8 | 1.8 |
| 8. | Suicide | 12.7 | 1.5 |
| 9. | Chronic liver disease and cirrhosis | 10.8 | 1.2 |
| 10. | Atherosclerosis | 9.2 | 1.1 |
| 11. | Nephritis, nephrotic syndrome & nephrosis | 9.1 | 1.0 |
| 12. | Homicide | 8.7 | 1.0 |
| 13. | Septicemia | 8.2 | 0.9 |
| 14 | Certain conditions in the perinatal period | 7.5 | 0.9 |
| 15. | Human immunodeficiency virus infection | 5.5 | 0.6 |
| All other causes | | 115.4 | 13.2 |

SOURCE: Based on National Center for Health Statistics data.

patients, if the disease were viewed in perspective. This is why I have discussed various aspects of the AIDS issue in such detail so far. I believe all people should try to learn as much as possible about AIDS to improve their understanding of the disease. We should then view AIDS as a "regular" disease that happens to kills its victims, just as heart disease, cancer, stroke, and the like are killer diseases. We should look at AIDS as a disease that can be contracted by anybody. We should view AIDS in the bigger scheme of things; that is, it should be viewed in relation to other diseases in terms of life and money lost.

Table 7.1 displays the 15 leading causes of death in the United States for 1987, the latest year for which data were available by fall 1990. It is clear that AIDS is not one of the top killer diseases; it ranks 15 out of 15. Remarkably, such "benign" diseases as pneumonia/influenza, diabetes, and cirrhosis kill more people in the United States than AIDS. If one considers the fact that the United States leads all nations in the number of reported AIDS cases, one can put the AIDS epidemic into global perspective. In every country of the world from which AIDS cases have been reported, AIDS does not rank as a leading cause of death. Even in African countries, the death rate from AIDS is lower than from such conditions as tuberculosis, measles, and diarrheal diseases.

These facts are not meant to minimize the seriousness and devastation of the AIDS epidemic. AIDS is a very serious disease because it is so complex and fatal. I would still consider it serious even if it killed only 100 people worldwide. Even more serious is its potential to become a leading cause of death, particularly in some African countries. It has the *potential* to kill millions of people rapidly. What is clear is that AIDS is not easily contracted, and it is not *currently* killing millions of people; it should not be feared in those terms. There is potential for this fear to lead to hopelessness and the temptation to write off AIDS/HIV-infected people and some populations. AIDS has to be viewed in perspective for the development of strategies to combat it.

Regarding black people and AIDS, it should be clear that they seem to be more affected not because of genetic reasons but because of environmental, especially socioeconomic, reasons. It should be clear that the high rates of AIDS cases in blacks reflect a high rate of poverty among blacks, whether in the United States, Haiti, or Africa. It should be clear that, in absolute numbers and by the percentage of the total number of AIDS cases in the United States, more whites have AIDS and have died from AIDS than blacks. In other words, blacks have a *disproportionately* high rate of AIDS based on their representation in the U.S. population. But something needs to be done so that the disproportion does not get wider.

So what should be done about AIDS among black people? First, the situation should be viewed in perspective. The disease of AIDS—its distribution in different populations, its transmission, and its pathogenesis—should be understood. It should then be understood that AIDS is not a genetic disease. Plans should then be developed to combat the problem, and they should be developed in a comprehensive manner. One cannot, and should not, address the issue of AIDS in blacks without taking into consideration their overall health status, which is greatly influenced by their socioeconomic status.

# REFERENCES

Gostlin, L. D. (1989). Public health strategy for confronting AIDS. *JAMA, 261,* 1621-1630.

Skattery, M. L., Robison, L. M., et al. (1989). Cigarette smoking and exposure to passive smoking are risk factors to cervical cancer. *JAMA, 261,* 1598.

U.S. Department of Health and Human Services. (1981). *Promoting health/preventing disease: Objectives for the nation, 1990.* Washington, DC: Government Printing Office.

Wake, W. T. (1989, March 20). How many patients will die because we fear AIDS? *Medical Economics,* pp. 24-30.

Warner, K. E. (1985). Cigarette advertising and media coverage of smoking and health. *The New England Journal of Medicine, 312,* 384-388.

Warner, K. E. (1989). Smoking and health: 25-year perspective. *American Journal of Public Health, 79,* 141-143.

Wilde, H. (1989). Cigarette export promotion by the American government. *The New England Journal of Medicine, 320,* 600.

# 8

## Control of the AIDS Epidemic: A Comprehensive Approach

The United States and, indeed, the world have traditionally responded to epidemics with a comprehensive approach. This has included such measures as quarantine, isolation, vaccination, and treatment. These traditional measures have been supplemented by research and education. The comprehensive approach has largely been successful in controlling most epidemics. Success has usually been achieved when most of the measures mentioned above were employed. The plague, yellow fever, and cholera control are examples of such successes. And, of course, the eradication of smallpox was through a well-organized comprehensive approach to epidemic control.

Control of epidemics is less successful when the measures used rely on individual behavior modification. In this regard, efforts by the U.S. Centers for Disease Control and the World Health Organization to control syphilis, gonorrhea, and other sexually transmitted diseases have not been very successful. Neither has there been a lot of success in controlling heart disease, cancer, and other so-called diseases of civilization through prevention. The control of AIDS is and will be difficult because the transmission of HIV involves mostly personal behavior—behavior that is well entrenched and involves psychosocial and cultural beliefs. These beliefs are difficult to change, particularly regarding a disease as controversial as AIDS.

As discussed in Chapter 4, the process of transmission of HIV and the pathogenesis of AIDS make AIDS potentially fully preventable. However, because of the relative uniqueness of the transmission and pathogenesis, some of the traditional measures of epidemic control

120

such as quarantine and isolation would not work. Even education at the mass level is not likely to be very effective in controlling AIDS. The control of AIDS should, therefore, involve *special comprehensive* programs. It should take into consideration the special characteristics and needs of AIDS/HIV-infected patients. It should consider individual and population characteristics.

Education is obviously the best tool (if not the only tool) currently available to control the AIDS epidemic. Education should be comprehensive; it should cover research, treatment, and prevention. For education to be successful, the individual and the community must be understood. Health status, particularly in terms of socioeconomic health, should be understood. And, before plans can be developed to control AIDS in any population, the impact of the disease should be reassessed.

## THE IMPACT OF AIDS ON SOCIETY

In raw numbers, AIDS is not a leading disease in terms of morbidity and mortality in most countries. Some countries have not even reported AIDS cases. Yet the devastation of AIDS affects all nations and all people of the world. The newness of AIDS, its complex nature in terms of transmission and pathogenesis, its almost universal fatality, and the fact that it has no cure make it a disease that affects many aspects of human existence. Knowledge of AIDS is evolving, and the full impact of AIDS on society is yet to be realized.

### Demographic Impact

The number of lives AIDS has claimed worldwide in a relatively short time is rather alarming. Tens of thousands of people have AIDS or have died from it since its discovery. Even more alarming is the number of people believed to be infected with HIV worldwide. Some populations are particularly hard hit; homosexuals, black Americans, and some black Africans are disproportionately affected.

Perhaps the most distressing aspect is the age group affected. Most AIDS illness and death have occurred in young people in the prime of their lives, their most economically productive years. In some parts of Africa, the future of entire nations is threatened because the future leaders are now the most affected by AIDS. If effective control measures are not instituted, populations with disproportionately high AIDS/HIV-infection cases are going to be diminished in size. If effective control measures are not instituted, populations not yet much affected are going to have many more cases and deaths.

## The Human Impact

As stated in earlier chapters, no disease in recent history has stirred and continues to stir so much fear and anxiety as AIDS. Both victims and healthy citizens react to the disease with fear. Even in countries where few or no cases of AIDS have been reported, the reaction is the same. AIDS seems to have an impact on all citizens of the world.

Family members of AIDS patients may have to contend with the stigma of someone whose life-style may not be socially acceptable. They may have to deal with a sick adult or child who grows increasingly dependent for physical and emotional support. Their finances may be exhausted rather quickly. The end result may be desertion or abandonment of the patients. The number of AIDS children and even some adults left in big city hospitals by their families are a testimony to this fact. There may be family disintegration. Friends may become instant counselors and the main source of physical and emotional support.

Employers may have to grapple with protecting an AIDS patient's or HIV-infected person's right to privacy and employment versus other employees' fear of contracting the virus. School officials may have to deal with the same situation for employees and students. In addition to the somewhat indirect way all citizens are affected by AIDS, if current trends continue, most people will know someone with AIDS in the next 10 years.

AIDS patients have to contend with a chronic debilitating disease. They have to endure pain from cancer or recurrent opportunistic infections. Chronic disease leads to weight loss and decreased energy levels. Debilitation leads to an inability to work. Patients tend to lose their jobs because they are too sick to work or because of job discrimination. Patients tend to lose insurance policies after losing their jobs; they may lose housing because of inability to pay rent or mortgage or because of housing discrimination. The end result may be reliance on public support by AIDS patients for housing, health care, counseling, and help with activities of daily living.

**Financial Impact**

I stated in Chapter 7 that the financial cost of AIDS to society is lower than that of several other diseases. But the cost as it relates to the number of cases is quite substantial; that is, the cost of research, education, and medical care is disproportionately higher than for other diseases. Studies in the United States indicate that costs for AIDS patients from diagnosis to death range from $50,000 to $140,000 per case. These are only health care costs, depending upon whether most of the care is provided in a hospital or home setting. Because of loss of jobs and insurance, most AIDS patients require public assistance for the medical and other services discussed above. In addition to their need for public assistance, the contribution by most AIDS patients to their countries' economies is lost. Most current AIDS patients are in their most economically productive years; they tend to be relatively well educated and possess good jobs.

The financial impact of AIDS is even more burdensome in Third World nations, particularly some African countries. Many of these countries had been struggling to control other diseases with inadequate finances before AIDS arrived. Not only has AIDS added much more to health care financial need, it has affected whole economies by claiming economically productive citizens. Some of these countries have been trying to control AIDS to the detriment of battling other diseases.

As stated at the beginning of this section, the full impact of AIDS on society is not known. However, it is obvious that the current impact is substantial enough to demand sound strategic planning. The demographic, human, and financial impact of AIDS make it one of the most costly diseases. Ironically, medical costs are likely to increase as more drugs are discovered to treat AIDS and as patients live longer. I believe the world has the capacity to control AIDS despite the seemingly prohibitive price tag. Indeed, the world has no choice but to move quickly to control this devastating disease.

## STRATEGIC PLAN TO CONTROL THE AIDS EPIDEMIC

The goal of controlling an epidemic is twofold: (a) to improve the condition of those with the disease and (b) to prevent those without the disease from getting it. The overall approach should be one of prevention; that is, primary prevention to ensure that those not exposed to HIV remain free of exposure, secondary prevention to ensure that those infected do not progress to AIDS, and tertiary prevention to ensure that AIDS patients live as long and healthy a life as possible. The plan should have four programs: (a) services to people with AIDS and HIV infection, (b) testing and counseling, (c) research, and (d) education.

## Services to People With AIDS and HIV Infection

It should be clear by now that people with AIDS require many different kinds of services. The impact of the disease on patients is so profound that even the strongest, wealthiest, and best adjusted individual can be reduced to a helpless soul. Very high medical costs, lost jobs, and sometimes lost housing contribute to the destitution of many AIDS patients.

*Medical care.* Despite aggressive research, there is no cure or effective treatment for HIV. The only drug approved to treat AIDS is Zidovidine (formerly AZT). As discussed in Chapter 4, AZT kills HIV in vitro (in the test tube). It works by preventing the multiplication of HIV. Therefore, it theoretically should be a cure for AIDS. Since its approval in 1987, its use has prolonged the lives of some AIDS patients, but it has severe side effects that limit its use. It is also very expensive, costing as much at $10,000 for one year of treatment.

Because there is no cure for HIV, AIDS patients spend a lot of time in the hospital for recurrent infections and are in and out of hospitals for treatment. Because their immune systems are destroyed, infections that are usually cured by antibiotics with the help of the immune system are only temporarily halted. In a few months, sometimes a few weeks, after leaving the hospital, the infections are reactivated, and the patients are back in the hospital. Some of the infections, for example *Pneumocyctis carinii* pneumonia (PCP) are difficult to treat. The offending organisms often develop resistance to the usual antibiotics, and other antibiotics have to be used. In the case of PCP, trimethoprim/sulfamethoxazole is often substituted for the usual Pentamidine, which is quite toxic.

The use of AZT is limited by its toxicity; that is, some of the toxic side effects can accelerate the death of AIDS patients. However, many patients have benefited and have lived longer by using AZT. It has been particularly beneficial when used in combination with other antiviral agents such as Interferon. But, because of the very high cost of using AZT, many AIDS patients are unable to use it at all or long enough time. There are many experimental drugs being used to treat HIV. Here again, not all those needing these drugs are being reached. The end result of no effective treatment for HIV is recurrent infections requiring frequent hospital stays—a very expensive proposition.

The strategic plan regarding medical care should ensure that all those needing AZT should get it regardless of income status. Experimental protocols should reach all eligible individuals. This may be difficult to accomplish because most experiments take place at medical schools and other research centers; patients living far from such centers may not know about the protocols. Every effort should be made to reach as many AIDS patients as possible for experimental drug treatment. In this regard, the federal government's recently announced (May 1989) hot line for new drug information is laudable. Anyone can call a toll-free number (1-800-TRIALS-A) and be informed of what experimental drugs are available in which locations for AIDS patients.

Drug treatment for asymptomatic HIV infection has been even more tenuous. Without a safe and effective drug to arrest the propagation of HIV, most people with HIV infection would ultimately progress to AIDS. AZT would be an excellent drug to prevent progression to AIDS but its intolerable side effects have precluded its use for such purposes. As safer antiviral agents are being tested, every effort should be made to keep HIV-infected people as healthy as possible. Strategic planning here should involve close medical follow-up testing for the number and quality of lymphocytes. Patients should be provided with adequate nutrition, stress management, and proper exercise to maximize their health status. They should avoid sexually transmitted and other cofactor diseases. They should be checked often and promptly treated for such diseases.

When AZT was approved in 1987 for the treatment of AIDS, its use was limited to adults with severe AIDS symptomatology because of its toxic side effects. A dose of 1,200 milligrams (mg) per day was used. In an attempt to reduce toxicity, lower doses were tried, and it has been concluded that 500 mg per day is as effective as 1,200 mg with many fewer side effects. Obviously, the lower dose has other benefits also, such as cost. This will allow many more AIDS patients to use AZT when resources are limited. More important, the lower dose, with its attendant fewer side effects, permits its use in HIV-infected patients without AIDS symptoms.

In 1990, the AIDS Clinical Trial Group (ACTG) Proticol 019 demonstrated beneficial effects of the lower dose of AZT in HIV-infected people. Subsequently, the Food and Drug Administration (FDA) approved AZT for this purpose. Because even the lower dose is not without side effects, not all HIV-infected people should use AZT. The ACTG recommendation is that individuals with a T4 lymphocyte count of less than 500 should be treated with AZT to prevent progression to clinical AIDS. In an article published in the October 1990 issue of *The New England Journal of Medicine* (Collier, 1990), researchers in California reported that doses even lower than 500 mg are effective. This, of course, is good news—lower dose means lower cost and more people being reached. Other antiretroviral drugs are being studied. Some of these are believed to have fewer side effects than AZT.

AZT prevents the multiplication of the virus, thus halting the destruction of lymphocytes and reversing the disease process. Therefore, a person testing positive for HIV antibodies should be tested for lymphocyte count. If the T4 count is less than 500, AZT should be offered; if more than 500, a lymphocyte count should be done every six months.

In addition to preventing lymphocyte destruction, prevention of opportunistic infections is recommended. The U.S. Public Health Service has published guidelines for preventive treatment of PCP. As mentioned before, trimethoprim/sulfamethoxazole (TMP-SMX) and Pentamidine are used to treat PCP; they are the same drugs recommended for preventive treatment (prophylaxis). One double-strength capsule a day of TMP-SMX or aerolized Pentamidine is recommended for prophylaxis. Aerolized Pentamidine goes directly into the lungs and very little is absorbed, thus leading to very few side effects in this regard; 150 mg once every two weeks or 300 mg once every four weeks of aerolized Pentamidine is recommended. Prophylaxis is recommended for individuals with T4 counts less than 200.

In 1990, the FDA approved Investigational New Drug (IND) status for AZT for children with HIV infection. IND status allows the distribution of a drug not yet approved for general use by any U.S. physician for serious and life-threatening diseases. Like other experimental protocols, treatment IND tends to be more available at medical schools and other major medical centers.

*Home care.* There are two major problems with medical care of AIDS patients: (a) There is no effective treatment for HIV and (b) the treatment of recurrent infections is very expensive. A comprehensive strategic plan is needed to approach these problems. As research on new and safer drugs goes on, alternatives to frequent hospital stay should be sought. Outpatient facilities should be expanded for AIDS-related services so that some inpatient services can be provided at less cost. Home health care programs should be instituted; services should include skilled nursing care, social work, occupational and physical therapy, nutritional services, and help in activities of daily living. Every effort should be made to keep AIDS patients out of the hospital as much as possible.

*General counseling.* A devastating disease like AIDS carries with it many problems that require counseling. The burden of chronic illness, lost relationships, lost housing, lost jobs, and lost insurance all lead to stress and require counseling. Services should include peer counseling, pastoral counseling by appropriate religious figures, and counseling with social workers, physicians, and psychologists. These services, which are mainly to enhance emotional well-being, should be supplemented by other services such as financial and legal counseling. These latter services should provide counseling on housing, discrimination, and confidentiality issues as well as eligibility for governmental and private assistance programs.

*Hospice care.* Because AIDS is an incurable condition, the issue of death is an ever-present concern for AIDS patients and their families. Hospice care has been useful to many AIDS patients and their families to deal with the issue of dying. Hospice programs should be available in communities so AIDS patients can avail themselves of the precious services hospice provides. Referrals may be made by physicians, hospitals, and families. Here again, pastoral and other forms of counseling should be available in addition to medicines for pain control.

## Testing and Counseling

A major factor in the control of the AIDS epidemic is identification of those infected with HIV. The purpose here is primary and secondary prevention: primary prevention so that individuals testing positive may not expose others to the virus; secondary prevention so that those testing positive may practice certain behaviors and receive prophylactic treatment to prevent their progressing to AIDS.

The most widely used tests for HIV infection are the ELISA and Western Blot tests to detect antibodies to HIV. The tests have been

available since June 1985 and, since their adoption, the CDC has recommended that testing be accompanied by pre- and posttest counseling. Indeed, testing without counseling is useless and may be
counterproductive because of the unique characteristics of HIV infection. The individual being tested should understand fully what the test
is supposed to detect, and he or she should clearly understand what
negative and positive antibody results mean.

As discussed in Chapter 4, there could be a "lag" period of more
than six months from HIV infection to development of antibodies.
Therefore, a person testing negative for HIV antibodies may actually
be infected. It is imperative that the person testing negative fully understand the lag period and modify behavior accordingly. The issue of
false positive tests should also be discussed. For this reason, taking a
thorough personal history during pretest counseling is important.
When the test is deemed to be a true positive, counseling should be
provided on proper nutrition, stress management, proper exercise and
rest, and avoidance of STDs and other cofactor diseases. The individual should be quickly placed into some health care system if he or
she does not already have a regular physician. He or she should be
followed regularly for checkup and treatment of all diseases likely to
effect progression to AIDS. He or she should also periodically have
lymphocyte counts. The need for all these follow-up activities should
be fully explained during posttest counseling sessions.

To be most effective, a testing and counseling service should be
both available and accessible. Ideally, the whole population should be
tested for HIV antibodies. Obviously, this is not practical, and the
consensus is that people in high-risk groups should be tested. In this
regard, it is recommended that homosexuals and heterosexuals with
multiple sexual partners, IV drug users, prostitutes, people attending
STD clinics, hospital inpatients, and pregnant women be tested. Regardless of who gets tested, the main issue is availability and accessi-
bility. Testing facilities should be available in communities, and the
cost should be low enough (or free) so that anybody needing testing
can have it. Above all, the testing facilities should have trained personnel who are knowledgeable, compassionate, and nonjudgmental to
serve the people needing testing. Absolute confidentiality should be
maintained at all testing centers.

A partner notification program is extremely important in the control of HIV infection. During posttest counseling, names, addresses,
and telephone numbers of all needle sharing and sexual partners

should be obtained. The clients should be assured that their names will not be used. They should be given the option of notifying the partners but the notification should not be left up to them. They should encourage their partners to come for testing. If they are unwilling to do the notification or if partners do not show up for testing within a reasonable time period, the testing agency should trace the contacts.

Contact tracing should be in the form of a letter, phone call, or visit. Whatever form it takes, the message should be simple and not reveal the condition to be tested or the original client's identity. For example: "We have information that you have been exposed to a serious communicable disease. Please call or come by as soon as possible." It may take several letters, phone calls, or visits, but every effort should be made to get partners tested and counseled. If the testing agent does not have personnel to do contact tracing, the information should be turned over to the local health department for tracing.

## Research

Research is important in the control of any epidemic; it is particularly necessary for the AIDS epidemic in that knowledge on the disease continues to evolve. A lot of research is going on in many parts of the world on vaccine development, new drugs, and basic science. These should continue at full speed. However, it is obvious that we cannot wait until an effective vaccine and drugs are developed in order to control the epidemic. Other control measures than vaccine and drugs require epidemiological studies.

As stated at the beginning of this chapter, a comprehensive program to control the AIDS epidemic should be community based. It is necessary, therefore, to have a reasonably accurate idea of the number of individuals infected with the virus in a community; prevalence studies are a means to achieve this. Most data currently available on HIV infection are obtained from individuals who voluntarily seek testing. These individuals may be involved in behaviors that place them at higher risk for HIV infection, and their test results may not be representative of their communities. On the other hand, some people involved in high-risk behaviors may not get tested.

In addition to the groups listed in the last section, all newborns, clients attending family planning clinics, TB patients, and selected students may be tested. Testing for prevalence studies should be confidential and anonymous; that is, while pre- and posttest counseling may occur, the results should not be reported with the individuals' names. However, demographic data such as race, sex, age, area of residence, and other behavioral characteristics should be reported. Again, the purpose of prevalence studies is to have an accurate idea of the HIV-infection rate in a community to plan control measures more appropriately.

As important as or perhaps more important than prevalence studies are surveillance studies. It is generally accepted that AIDS and HIV-infection cases are underreported worldwide. This is because most reports are based on passive surveillance; that is, agencies diagnosing AIDS or HIV-antibody positivity voluntarily report to local health authorities. When authorities do not receive reports, it is assumed that no cases have been diagnosed in the particular community, which, of course, could be a false assumption. A comprehensive AIDS control program should include an active surveillance component. There should be a surveillance specialist(s) with direct contact with physicians, hospitals, clinics, and laboratories in the community to collect up-to-date data on AIDS and HIV-antibody diagnosis.

A third component of epidemiological studies is one involving disease association. Current data clearly demonstrate increased incidence of TB in people with AIDS and HIV infection. Research here should involve testing all newly diagnosed TB patients for HIV and doing TB skin tests on all those testing positive for HIV antibodies. Also, preliminary data indicate an association between HIV infection and severe syphilis (neurosyphilis). The indication is that, in the presence of HIV infection, primary syphilis progresses very quickly to neurosyphilis without the usual preceding secondary and tertiary stages. Furthermore, neurosyphilis in the presence of HIV infection usually does not respond to the typical penicillin therapy. People with neurosyphilis or any stage of syphilis not responding to conventional therapy should be tested for HIV antibodies. Research on the association between HIV infection and these two diseases will shed better light on the extent of HIV infection in the community. In addition, it should help in the development of a better treatment plan for TB and syphilis. Obviously, research on the association between HIV infection and other diseases should be conducted.

## Education

Without a doubt, education is the best tool to control the AIDS epidemic as there remains no cure or vaccine for the disease. Modification of population and individual characteristics through education is the only means of controlling the spread of HIV. Education on AIDS has two purposes: (a) to alleviate unreasonable fears about AIDS and (b) to prevent the spread of HIV. Both purposes require dissemination of accurate, up-to-date, and understandable information about AIDS and HIV infection. To be effective, an educational message should be consistent, persuasive, and repeated often. Again, an AIDS education program should be comprehensive and community based.

*Public information.* Telephone lines should be available in designated local health agencies for people to call with specific inquiries. The telephones obviously should be manned by trained personnel well acquainted with all aspects of the AIDS issue. The personnel should be multilingual when community demographics warrant it. Public service announcements on television and radio should frequently be made. Articles on AIDS should frequently appear in local newspapers in appropriate community languages. Public service announcements and newspaper articles should not simply give facts or report new findings but should provide understandable and useful information. Media personnel should be well educated on AIDS to provide needed education to the public.

"AIDS libraries" should be set up in local libraries, local health agencies, schools, hospitals, and community centers. Printed, audio, and video material in appropriate community languages should be available to impart understandable and useful information. The material should always contain information on where to go for further information. Community forums and symposia should be frequently held during which experts, preferably from the community, are invited to discuss various aspects of the AIDS issue.

*Workplace AIDS education.* The major issue of AIDS in the workplace involves the rights of AIDS and HIV-infected patients to employment versus the fear of other employees' contracting the virus. Another issue is some health workers' reluctance to take care of AIDS patients. In both situations, education should be directed at alleviating unreasonable fears and outlining measures to prevent exposure to blood and body fluids. Employers in both public and private agencies should have periodic conferences in which experts can speak to employees on AIDS. Selected employees should be trained to be resource persons to provide ongoing education. Experts should be invited to discuss legal, personnel, and insurance issues. Workplace AIDS policy, including infection control protocol, should be developed jointly by employers, employees, and experts. The policy should periodically be updated as new information on AIDS becomes available. Finally, employers should make safety equipment available if a chance exists at the workplace for exposure to blood and body fluids.

*School AIDS education.* The situation in educational institutions regarding AIDS is more complex. It involves development of workplace policy and curricula to provide information about AIDS. Workplace policy here involves protection of the rights of AIDS/HIV-infected employees to work and AIDS/HIV-infected students to attend school. Education of employees and prevention of exposure to blood and other body fluids should be accomplished as described above.

Schools and universities are the most likely sites for effective primary prevention of AIDS. Children and young adults in educational institutions have the potential to experiment with sexual and drug use behaviors that put them at risk for AIDS. Education on AIDS, therefore, should be part of a comprehensive system to modify these behaviors. There has been controversy about how early in the school system sexual matters should be discussed. Former U.S. Surgeon General C. Everett Koop suggested that AIDS should be taught at the lowest grade possible. I believe that the community should decide which grade level is appropriate for teaching about AIDS. Regardless of what grade level at which a community decides to start AIDS education, instruction should involve all three levels of educational institutions—elementary, secondary, and university.

As part of a comprehensive program, instruction on HIV infection should include the biology of HIV infection in terms of simple virology, genetics, transmission, pathogenesis, and treatment. Behaviors that affect transmission and pathogenesis should be discussed, and modification of these behaviors should be emphasized. Particular attention should be paid to individual responsibility regardless of how young the student may be. Obviously, the level of technical and frank sexual language used in the classroom will depend upon the grade level, but discussion should be detailed enough for full understanding.

The aim of a comprehensive AIDS educational program should be health promotion and disease prevention. Therefore, the curriculum should contain materials on other sexually transmitted diseases, drug use, tobacco and alcohol use, teenage pregnancy, and proper nutrition and exercise. The curriculum should be progressive; that is, knowledge at one grade level should be built upon at succeeding grade levels. And the curriculum should be periodically revised as new information becomes available. Teachers should be properly trained in all aspects of the curriculum; they should have periodic in-service training to update their knowledge. Guest speakers from the health professions should be invited periodically to speak to students and other school employees.

*AIDS education in special populations.* The different educational approaches discussed above should reach all segments of society if efficiently implemented. However, certain groups may require special attention in dealing with their particular needs in AIDS prevention. Homosexual/bisexual men, IV drug users, prostitutes, and people with physical and emotional handicaps should be targeted for special AIDS education. Again, the aim should be to promote overall good health.

Homosexual activity is the biggest risk behavior of HIV transmission and pathogenesis into AIDS in many countries. It also promotes other sexually transmitted viral and bacterial diseases. Homosexual and bisexual men should be taught the same biological and behavioral components for HIV and the other infections. In addition, their specific sexual practices—that is, penile-anal sex, "fisting," introduction of inanimate objects into the rectum, and multiple sexual partnership—should be discussed in relation to how they promote disease. Lectures and discussions may occur at various community settings, including gay bars, bathhouses, and arcades.

IV drug users are particularly difficult to reach with education involving behavior change. However, they represent the biggest threat to the spread of AIDS in many developed countries, and any AIDS control program without attention to IV drug use will not be maximally effective. Many IV drug users do not voluntarily seek education because of the illicit nature of their behavior. The focus of AIDS education, therefore, should be on drug use itself. Drug treatment centers should be set up in communities, preferably in existing structures such as hospitals, community centers, and churches. Jails and prisons are also good places to institute drug treatment and AIDS education. As part of teaching to refrain from IV drug use and the sharing of needles, HIV and other infections should be discussed. Emphasis should be placed on the role of needle sharing and unprotected sexual activity in the spread of various diseases.

Prostitutes also are difficult to reach because their activity is illegal in many countries. But they need to be reached because of the risks involved in their practice. Many prostitutes also use illicit drugs, at least in developed countries, and can be reached through drug treatment facilities. Also in some countries, a large portion of jail and prison inmates are prostitutes; education in jails and prisons should reach them.

There are no data on the number of AIDS cases among people with physical and mental disability, although the number seems to be low. However, because of their special needs, every effort should be made to prevent the spread of HIV in that population. Written material should be made available in Braille for the blind, sign language interpretation should be available at lecture/discussion sessions, TDD (telephone device for the deaf) equipment should be provided at telephone information services, and staff at mental institutions should be especially trained to prevent exchange of blood and other body fluids among patients.

Inmates of jails and prisons often carry communicable diseases at admission, and life behind bars puts them at risk for other communicable diseases. Homosexual activity and illicit drug use occur quite frequently, even in those who did not indulge in such activities on the outside. Prisons provide a good opportunity for health education given that the inmates are a captive audience. They may have no place to go or nothing to do and thus be "forced" to attend lecture/discussions on health issues. Perhaps a better approach would be a regularly scheduled time period for health education. Inmates would be encouraged, instead of forced, to attend. The classes should be interesting and practical enough that inmates would find them beneficial. Many of them might attend just to break the boredom of prison life but may later enjoy and learn something if the classes are well organized. Inmates may be asked to be guest speakers; others may be involved in role-playing. Discussion of HIV infection should be supplemented by that of other diseases, nutrition and exercise, stress management, and job counseling to encourage inmates to stay out of prison.

Finally, the use of alcohol should be discussed in conjunction with AIDS education at all levels. Alcohol impairs judgment and may lead to irresponsible sexual behavior or needle sharing. People may indulge in sexual activity more readily when they are drunk than when they are sober. Also, people who use condoms consistently may not use them when they are drunk. Responsible use of alcohol (or complete abstinence) makes for good overall health maintenance. Young people particularly need to be educated on the responsible use of alcohol.

## CONCLUSION

I have discussed a strategic plan to control the AIDS epidemic on the basis of four programs, but they are not mutually exclusive. A successful control program should be comprehensive and thus simultaneously provide the services discussed above. This requires careful planning, which may have to involve many agencies and different funding sources. The important thing is that it should be community based—members of the community should be part of planning and implementing programs.

Obviously, services to people with AIDS and HIV infection may not be necessary in communities without cases. However, a comprehensive plan should include such services and provisional budgets should be made. Hopefully, other programs would be so effective that the community would remain free of AIDS cases; but, if cases do occur, the community would be ready to provide the necessary services. It should be recognized that AIDS does not occur only in certain geographic areas or risk groups. The whole world has been and will continue to be affected by AIDS; the control of the epidemic, therefore, depends upon worldwide effort.

## REFERENCE

Collier, A. C. (1990). A pilot study of low-dose zidovudine in human immunodeficiency virus infection. *The New England Journal of Medicine, 323,* 1015-1021.

# 9

## The Control of AIDS in Black Populations: The Comprehensive Approach

> Improved health owes less to advances in medical science than to changes in the external environment and to a favorable trend in the standard of living. . . . We are healthier than our ancestors not because of what happens when we are ill, but because we do not become ill.
>
> —World Health Organization (1957)

I stated in Chapters 1 and 6 that the prevalence of AIDS is disproportionately high in black populations for the same reasons that the prevalence of other diseases is higher. Their overall health status is lower, so they are prone to all sorts of diseases. Their overall health status is lower because of their generally overall lower socioeconomic status. Therefore, plans to control AIDS in blacks should address their overall health and socioeconomic status. The WHO declaration quoted above should serve as the backbone of the control effort.

Examples were given in Chapter 6 regarding the effect of changes in the external environment and a favorable trend in the standard of living. Many black people in both developed and developing countries enjoy a relatively poor external environment and standard of living. Some of them are not much healthier than their ancestors, and it is they who are afflicted most by *all kinds of diseases* including AIDS. Furthermore, the modest advances in the treatment of AIDS have largely missed them. Black people are less likely to be treated with AZT and other experimental drugs; and African blacks are even less likely to participate in those treatment protocols. Indeed, blacks have been less involved in all four programs of the strategic plan; they are less likely to be involved in testing and counseling, research, and educational programs.

An exception to the lack of experimental drug protocol in blacks is the use of oral Interferon in Kenya. Interferon is a natural substance produced by the body to fight all kinds of viruses. Synthetic Interferon has been used on an experimental basis for many years to treat certain cancers; it has also been used in this manner to treat genital warts. Various researchers have tried intravenous Interferon, with some success, to treat AIDS. This work with Interferon has mainly been done at research centers with relatively few patients. The intravenous route makes it more expensive and less practical in terms of reaching AIDS patients. Therefore, a pill form that is relatively inexpensive is much needed to reach many more patients.

Kemron is a low-dose synthetic Interferon in pill form consisting of different forms of alpha-Interferon. It was developed by a U.S. company but produced by a Japanese company. It was used by the Kenya Medical Research Institute to treat AIDS patients. After one year of experimental use, the Kenyan researchers reported very good results. The patients reported overall improvement in general well-being, improvement in appetite and weight gain, and improvement in strength. The researchers observed alleviation of symptoms and increased T4 counts. In July 1990, the Kenyan government approved the general use of Kemron to treat AIDS. By fall 1990, Kenya was the only country to approve Kemron for general use.

Kemron is not used in other countries purportedly because no other researchers than the Kenyan group have been able to duplicate the results of the Kenyan researchers. A WHO meeting in Geneva subsequent to Kemron approval in Kenya concluded that there was no conclusive evidence that low-dose oral Interferon was effective in treating AIDS.

## THE UNITED STATES

Black Americans are behind in the progress made toward the control of the AIDS epidemic partly due to the fact that the disease was initially viewed as a white homosexual disease. The black community in the United States initially denied the presence of the disease in blacks and the need to control it. Likewise, some black African governments initially denied the seriousness or even the presence of AIDS in their countries. Because of the denial and other reasons, black communities fell behind in the formation of community-based organizations and programs to control the epidemic. For example, the quite successful efforts of white homosexual support groups in providing various services to their members have been lacking in black communities. Even when it became clear that AIDS affects blacks, and that homosexual activity is the major risk behavior for HIV acquisition in blacks, they still do not have adequate participation in homosexually related activities/services.

In addition to being behind in the formation of community-based organizations to deal with the AIDS epidemic, the few organizations that have been formed have been unable to obtain funding from private sources such as foundations. Consequently, services to people with AIDS in black communities have depended upon government programs, which usually have rigid eligibility requirements and do not cover a large portion of individuals too poor to be included in funding for community-based testing and counseling, research, and education programs.

Perhaps what is most disappointing about the lack of community-based organizations in black communities is the absence of the leadership role of the black church. The church has historically been a positive force in black U.S. social and political life. It has been instrumental in most of the civil rights accomplishments by blacks. It has been looked upon for leadership in community activities. Unfortunately, this well-placed leadership role has not been utilized in the control of AIDS among black Americans. The black church has been reluctant to be involved in the AIDS issue because of the earlier misconception that AIDS is a white people's disease and the fact that homosexuals and IV drug users are most affected by the disease.

The reluctance of black churches to deal with AIDS stems from the view most churches have of AIDS. Because homosexual activity is viewed by many Christian believers as sin, some church leaders actually proclaimed at the beginning of the epidemic that AIDS is punishment for homosexual activity. To be associated with and help AIDS patients is to condone homosexuality. Some church leaders also perceive illicit drug use as a sin and would not advocate association with IV drug users with AIDS. The end result has been condemnation of AIDS patients in some cases and lack of support for the control effort in most cases. And the black community is missing a vital community resource.

Another community resource lacking in black communities is health professionals. As stated in the last chapter, community-sponsored symposia and forums should feature experts preferably from the local community. But black Americans are grossly underrepresented in the health professions. For example, only 2% of all U.S. physicians are black; the percentage of doctorate-level black scientists such as immunologists and epidemiologists is even lower. Recent data indicate that the number of black candidates applying for medical and other advanced science degrees has been decreasing.

There are many obstacles that have hampered progress in the establishment of community-based organizations to control the AIDS epidemic in black communities. However, trends are changing positively both in the United States and in developing nations. Efforts in the right direction should be continued and intensified. But a lot more remains to be done. Strategic planning is needed.

The general approach to strategic planning described in the last chapter should be employed in the control of the epidemic in black populations. However, social, cultural, language, and economic characteristics should be particularly emphasized in the implementation of programs. Available community resources should be utilized. When needed community resources are not available, they should be aggressively sought and utilized. Whole communities should be mobilized and made part of the control effort. The first step should be mobilization of community leadership through which programs could be effected.

The black church should be educated that AIDS is a disease that can affect anybody but, more important, affects blacks disproportionately. The church needs to understand that, whether or not AIDS is wrath from God on some sinners, its control is imperative lest it kill more "nonsinners." Then ministers and other church elders could provide valuable pastoral counseling. The church could be a gathering area for community symposia and forums. The church could carry out all sorts of fund-raising activities for the control effort. Church leaders could also approach politicians through their membership to influence local and national AIDS policy.

Other black organizations include political groups such as the NAACP, the Urban League, and the Southern Christian Leadership Conference; professional groups such as those of black police officers, lawyers, physicians, athletes, actors/actresses, musicians, and teachers; black newspaper and broadcast media personnel; and black student organizations on university campuses. These groups should be mobilized and educated on various aspects of the AIDS epidemic so that they can provide leadership in the control effort. Again, they are valuable resources for organizing symposia and forums and raising funds. Individuals in these groups may serve as role models for young blacks in overall health education; that is, some of these individuals would demonstrate close to ideal physical and socioeconomic health.

To repeat Admiral Watkins's proclamation: HIV has opened a window of opportunity to do something about the inadequate and maldistributed health care systems. Therefore, the strategic plan should be comprehensive and take other diseases in blacks into consideration. As stated several times in this book, there are so many cases of AIDS in blacks because there are so many other diseases stemming from their relatively low socioeconomic status. Control of AIDS cannot be maximally successful unless the whole health status is addressed. Therefore, testing and counseling, research, and education programs for AIDS should cover other "black" diseases. The approach is more likely to reach more people who might otherwise be less willing to participate in AIDS-related activities.

For example, a community clinic, instead of offering just HIV testing and counseling, may provide general screening. A whole family may visit the clinic where screening for hypertension, cancer, diabetes, sickle-cell disease, STD, and HIV would be done on various members of the family. Education would be provided as needed, and everyone would be educated on AIDS/HIV infection, proper nutrition and exercise, and avoidance of substance abuse including illicit drugs, cigarettes, and alcohol. Likewise, community presentations on AIDS/HIV infection should include discussion of other diseases. Health fairs may be part of cultural activities held in the community, during which screening and education on various diseases could be provided.

As stated earlier, not only are blacks disproportionately affected by AIDS, but black AIDS patients die more quickly from the disease. Studies have demonstrated that, while the overall average time from diagnosis to death is about 36 months, the average time for blacks is about 12 months. The reasons for quick death are not fully apparent but it seems to me there is not much mystery. The same reasons echoed throughout this book relate to quick death—poor overall health status, existence of cofactor diseases, lack of access to health care. Because of overall health status, HIV infection is likely to progress to AIDS more quickly. Cofactor diseases also contribute to quick progression to AIDS. And, because of lack of access (both physical and fiscal) to health care, the disease may be far advanced by the time medical care is sought.

Early diagnosis is key to moderating the high rates of quick death. Physicians and other health care providers should pay particular attention and offer HIV-antibody testing to susceptible blacks. Careful history taking to identify risk behavior/exposure is important. Once they test positive, people should be thoroughly educated on AIDS symptomatology. They should be immediately placed into a health care system for management of HIV infection. They should have T4 counts more frequently. They should be tested for cofactor diseases such as syphilis, TB, hepatitis, herpes, and cytomegalovirus. They should be educated on proper nutrition, exercise and rest, and stress management. Careful diet history should be taken, and diet recommendations should be individualized. The patients' home and work situations should be investigated such that appropriate meal substitutions could be made. For example, if the patient cannot afford or does not like meat, other sources of protein such as milk, nuts, peanut butter, and eggs could be recommended.

Every effort should be made to put them on AZT or other antiviral agents, as clinical status and T4 counts indicate. They should have access to experimental protocols as available. Arrangements for follow-up should be made; transportation should be provided as needed. Cofactor diseases should be aggressively treated; particular attention should be paid to syphilis and TB because the incidence of these two diseases is increasing with HIV infection and they also affect blacks disproportionately. Individuals should be placed on prophylaxis for PCP as described in the last chapter.

In addition to the cofactor diseases already discussed, another reason for quick progression to AIDS and quick death may be illicit drug use and prostitution. The use of crack cocaine is rather common in poor inner-city blacks. The drug itself has severe toxic effects on the body, which lead to poor health. Also, drug use behavior may facilitate needle sharing, poor nutrition, and prostitution (to exchange sex for drugs). The sex for drugs phenomenon is becoming a big problem in terms of HIV infection; it is believed to be a major reason of increasing HIV infection in black women and, consequently, a source of pediatric HIV infection. Recent data indicate that this phenomenon is spreading quickly to rural areas. Careful drug use and sexual history should be taken in STD, family planning, and prenatal clinics to identify those at risk of acquiring HIV through this phenomenon. Individuals should be educated on the need to use condoms. Counseling on drug use and prostitution should be offered as needed, and placement into drug treatment programs should be made appropriately.

A recent study published by the CDC (1990) on the use of condoms by heterosexuals found that blacks are less likely to use condoms. That same study showed that the use of condoms has contributed greatly to the decreased incidence of HIV infection in homosexuals in San Francisco. The use of condoms also helps to prevent other sexually transmitted diseases and unwanted pregnancy. Therefore, clients in the clinics mentioned above should be educated to use condoms and in the proper ways to use them.


## AFRICA

There are many more obstacles in the control of the epidemic among African blacks. In addition to those discussed above, language barriers, illiteracy, inadequate transportation, lack of clinic and hospital facilities, and inadequate testing equipment all hamper the control effort. Indeed, many of these obstacles have contributed to the historically poor health of many African blacks. The problems seem to have been ignored for years; now is the time to do something about them, seizing the window of opportunity opened by HIV.

A big obstacle is the inadequate number of trained health professionals in many African communities. In some areas, there are no African doctors or other health experts; medical care is provided by expatriates who usually do not speak the native language. In these cases, medical care is usually adequate if diagnosis and treatment are all that is involved; but, for patient education, language is extremely important. Both mass and one-on-one health education requires language that is understandable to the receivers of the message. Because behavior modification may be required in the control of the AIDS epidemic, one-on-one education is important. The educator and the educated must understand each other for the education to be effective.

Despite the obstacles, a lot can be and is being done in many African countries to improve the health of their citizens. The Kemron protocol in Kenya discussed earlier in this chapter is a good example. Another good example is the testing of vaccines in Zaire as discussed in Chapter 3. Many other countries have been using the concept of Primary Health Care (PHC) advocated by the World Health Organization to improve health.

The WHO (1982) defined PHC as "essential health care made . . . accessible to individuals and families in the community by means acceptable to them, through their full participation, and at a cost the community and the country can afford." The above definition of PHC originated at the Alma Ata Declaration of 1978 when the WHO designated PHC as the means to achieving "health for all by the year 2000." The WHO has identified eight essential services for PHC:

(1) health education

(2) food and nutrition

(3) water and sanitation

(4) maternal and child health

(5) expanded immunization

(6) control of communicable diseases

(7) treatment of disease and injury

(8) availability of essential drugs

Many African countries have embarked on PHC projects and made significant, albeit modest, progress in improving the health status of their citizens. Countries such as Ghana, Mali, Tanzania, and Zimbabwe have achieved significant progress. The PHC projects in these and other countries have been hampered by some of the obstacles discussed above plus extremely inadequate financial resources. Difficulties with primary health care implementation existed before the discovery of AIDS, and, obviously, AIDS has compounded the problem of health care in some African countries.

Regarding the control of the AIDS epidemic in Africa, the strategic plan discussed in the last chapter and above for U.S. blacks should be followed. However, it should be incorporated into a *special comprehensive* approach—that is, part of PHC implementation. The essential services of PHC as outlined above all apply to the control of the AIDS epidemic. In a presentation at the Fifth International Congress of the World Federation of Public Health Associations in Mexico

City, I proposed that health education be dropped as one of the essential services of PHC; instead, it should be part of each of the other seven services. The concept of PHC places emphasis on prevention of disease. I perceive health education as the backbone of prevention, to be utilized every step of the way in the prevention effort.

As stated above, there is a paucity of health professionals, particularly indigenous Africans, in many African countries. But the concept of PHC calls for the use of nonphysicians such as nurses and community health workers who are trained to provide basic medical and preventive services. Whether PHC services are provided by physicians or nonphysicians, language is paramount in providing effective education. It may be difficult to get the needed number of trained health professionals who speak the language of the community because many African countries have many different languages and dialects. In the presentation referred to above, I also proposed that schoolteachers should be trained and utilized in health education. Teachers are educators who should be able to present effective health education. Being established members of the community, they may be able to achieve easier rapport with the people they are educating. They are likely to speak the language or dialect of the community. When teachers teach students and members of the community, the consistency of the educational message is likely to be maintained; the chance of effecting behavior modification is enhanced by a consistent message.

Mass education involving electronic and print media is even more difficult because of the multiplicity of languages and high levels of illiteracy. Politicians have traditionally used posters, folklore, and song to get their messages across. These tools can be effectively utilized for health education messages. Programs should be developed locally by community leaders, and the contents should reflect local beliefs and tastes.

The lack of clinic and hospital facilities is a major problem in many African countries. Residents of some towns and villages may be as far as 100 miles from a hospital or clinic. And those available are often inadequately equipped and staffed. Existing facilities should be strengthened; mobile clinics should be made available in areas without clinics and hospitals. Also, "miniclinics" could be established in towns and villages with substandard transportation infrastructure. Existing buildings such as schools, churches, and community centers could be utilized. A room could be set up in these buildings to house portable kerosene-powered refrigerators for the storage of vaccines and other medicines and the room could also be used for storage of other nonperishable medicines and equipment. A trained resident would provide basic medical care at the miniclinic. The person or persons, of course, would be part of a multidisciplinary team providing comprehensive health services.

A school would be an ideal place for the "miniclinic." Many schools are strategically located so that most people can get to them on their way to work or the farm. And, of course, schoolchildren requiring primary care services would be right where the clinic is. Also, schools serve as the place for community activities in many African communities. Furthermore, if teachers are providing the bulk of the health services, it makes sense to have the clinic where the teachers are. Most people think of health in terms of disease; they might consider it more worthwhile to go for a vaccine or medicine and then also receive education on nutrition, water and sanitation, STDs and AIDS, and so on.

## CONCLUSION

The control of the AIDS epidemic is difficult and will remain difficult. It is even more difficult in black populations. Therefore, a well-planned, comprehensive approach should be followed. The task is great; obstacles abound; and the cost is tremendous. But the epidemic must be controlled.

Planners should understand the epidemiology, transmission, pathogenesis, and treatment of AIDS and HIV infection. They should understand the role of genetics and the environment in terms of the distribution of AIDS among different populations. The health status of U.S. blacks, as described in Chapter 2, and that of African blacks, as described in Chapter 5, should be taken into consideration. The AIDS epidemic should be viewed in perspective; it should be understood that AIDS is a disease that can affect anybody. People with AIDS and HIV infection should be given due sympathy and support and should not suffer from discrimination.

The theme of this book is that blacks have higher rates of AIDS because they are less healthy and poorer. The control of AIDS in blacks should, therefore, be coupled with the improvement of their overall health and economic status. The WHO has defined *health* as a state of complete physical mental and social well-being and not merely the absence of disease or infirmity. This WHO definition has been viewed as representing an unobtainable ideal. But it is clear that people who are healthy come closer to the definition. The goal then should be to approach this ideal state as much as possible. Plans to control the AIDS epidemic in blacks should provide for a state of physical, mental, social, and economic well-being.

## REFERENCES

Bolard, R. G. A., & Young, M. E. M. (1982). The strategy, costs, and progress of primary health care. *Bulletin of the Pan American Health Organization, 16,* 233-241.

Centers for Disease Control. (1990). Heterosexual behavior and factors that influence condom use among patients attending a sexually transmitted disease clinic: San Francisco. *MMWR, 39*(39), 685-689.

Morley, D. (1983). *Practicing health for all.* Oxford: Oxford University Press.

World Health Organization. (1948). *Constitution of the World Health Organization.* Geneva, Switzerland: Author.

World Health Organization. (1957). *World Health Organization Monograph No. 34.* Geneva, Switzerland: Author.

World Health Organization. (1982). *Health for all by the year 2000: Strategies.* Geneva, Switzerland: Author.

# 10

---

## Financing AIDS Control:
## It Can Be Done

The legitimate object of government is to do for a community of people whatever they need to have done but cannot do all in their separate and individual capacities.

—Abraham Lincoln

In many of my presentations, I outline strategies for the control of the AIDS epidemic. I have also been asked by businesses and governmental agencies to help them develop an AIDS control policy. In both situations, my ideas are accepted but I am often asked: Who will pay? Who should pay for the control of the AIDS epidemic? Can the world afford to pay the tremendous costs involved in the control of the epidemic? I believe a more appropriate question is this: Can the world afford *not* to pay? We simply have no choice but do what it takes to halt the spread of this devastating disease.

AIDS is a worldwide problem. It is a problem of governments, private businesses, charitable organizations; it is a problem of communities, families, individuals. The cost of controlling it, therefore, requires contributions from every sector of society. AIDS is everybody's problem, so everybody should contribute toward its control. Yet, one of the reasons the epidemic has spread so quickly is that appropriate contributions by responsible entities have not been made. Most appalling was the initially slow response of governments to financing AIDS research.

During the 1988 International Conference on AIDS in Stockholm, Sweden, I listened in dismay as Dr. Ruhakano Rugunda, former

Ugandan minister of health, lamented the lack of funds for international AIDS control projects. The WHO Global Program on AIDS had a budget of only $96 million for 1988. Member nations of WHO were not willing to give money to finance a "mere" $96 million budget; but the world's richest nations were spending *trillions* of dollars on arms—weapons of destruction—he said.

I was rather surprised by the relatively modest figure Dr. Rugunda gave, and I was also saddened that WHO was having difficulty raising the $96 million. Why is the WHO having difficulty raising this amount? I reminded myself that the problem is more political than economic. There is an economic slowdown in many countries, but there is enough money around that the WHO should be able to raise the needed funds. The WHO budget would mostly finance projects in countries where individual and governmental resources are inadequate. These countries have been chronically dependent on richer countries for all kinds of assistance. Historically, poor countries have had little trouble getting military assistance from the richer countries, but development projects have suffered chronically from lack of assistance.

The superpowers have used the poorer countries as political pawns in their race for military supremacy and often supply arms to acquire political alignment. By so doing, they endeavor to keep these countries dependent so they can be manipulated politically. Therefore, instead of sound long-term economic projects toward self-sufficiency, these countries are often given economic assistance in a crisis-oriented manner. For example, the devastating drought in Ethiopia went on for years and hundreds of people began to die before grain was sent from the richer countries.

To be sure, some of the poorer countries must share the blame. Corruption at the highest levels of government has contributed to the poor state of affairs in these countries. There are reports of government officials' and politicians' using foreign assistance money to build houses and swimming pools for themselves in some African countries. At times, even when the money is used as indicated, there is so much mismanagement that less than expected results are achieved.

The United States is the largest contributor to WHO, being responsible for about 25% of its budget. But, during most of the Reagan administration, the United States was behind in its contributions. The U.S. government also withheld funds from family planning projects by WHO purportedly because some of the funds would be used to promote abortion. This is the same government that promotes the sale of cigarettes to kill millions of people worldwide but is opposed to the so-called killing of unborn children. I must say that, as a physician, I am personally opposed to abortion; I have never performed one. But I believe it is shortsighted to withhold all funding for something as important as family planning because of one disputed issue. Population control is a key to the health, social, and economic development of many poor nations.

The Bush administration has continued to play politics with WHO funding. In May 1989, U.S. Secretary of State James Baker announced that the United States would cut funding to WHO if it accepted the Palestinian Liberation Organization (PLO) as a member. The U.S. government in effect held the health status of billions of people hostage for its own political gains. The WHO promptly denied PLO membership.

Such is the history of economic development in many poor nations. Both donor and recipient nations have played politics with development assistance. And the tradition has continued with the control of the AIDS epidemic. The sad thing is that thousands of people are dying because the world has lacked the political will to do what is necessary to control the epidemic.

The United States is in the best position to set a leadership example in the control effort. It has the largest number of AIDS cases in the world. It has the capacity to demonstrate ability to control the epidemic among its own people and assist the effort in other countries. But it has not shown such leadership. Though the United States currently spends more money than any other country on AIDS, the financial commitment has been very slow in coming. Necessary appropriations were not made at the initial stages of the epidemic. When substantial effort was initiated, the epidemic was quite well advanced, and funding appeared to be too little too late.

Subsequent attempts were more encouraging but recent developments indicate retrogression. The U.S. Congress enacted the Ryan White Comprehensive AIDS Resource Emergency Act to provide $880 million for AIDS prevention and treatment efforts. The act was in honor of Ryan White, the young hemophiliac who contracted AIDS through transfusion of clotting factors and died at age 18. Before the money was to be appropriated, it was reduced to $159 million during fiscal 1990-1991 budget negotiations. Also, a subcommittee of the Senate denied appropriation of $30 million to help AIDS patients buy AZT.

The lack of financial support is part of the overall lack of support for the whole AIDS issue. That is, because the populations initially affected were the "undesirables" of society, the sense of urgency governments usually attach to epidemics was not there. When President Nixon declared his so-called war on cancer and charged scientists to come up with a cure, he implied that money should not be an object. Nothing close to that commitment has been made by the U.S. government for AIDS. Even more disturbing is the fact that some scientists are complaining that AIDS is taking money and manpower away from other research activities.

It is encouraging that things have been improving in the United States in the last few years. The U.S. Congress has successively increased funding for AIDS. Many states are also committing substantial amounts of money. For example, the state of Texas, with the fourth highest number of reported AIDS cases among the 50 states, had allocated nothing for AIDS prior to 1987. The 1987-1988 legislature appropriated $1.8 million for the biennium, but the 1989-1990 legislature appropriated $18 million, mostly for education and prevention. Private agencies, foundations, and universities are spending millions of dollars on AIDS.

The laudable effort discussed above is not reaching many poor people, particularly poor black people. Black communities have not been successful in attracting funding from either governmental or private sources. The quotation from Abraham Lincoln at the opening of this chapter is particularly relevant to the black community. I stated earlier in the chapter that contributions for the control of the AIDS epidemic should come from every sector of society: Communities, families, individuals, and governments should all contribute substantially; then it is the object of government to do for the community what it cannot do for itself.

The inability to control the epidemic by communities is even more acute in Third World countries. Many of the African countries with high rates of AIDS cases are so economically destitute that not only can families and communities not contribute enough, the government cannot help substantially. The concept of Primary Health Care as defined by WHO calls for the provision of services "at a cost the community and the country can afford." AIDS has simply shattered the idea of community financing of PHC services. When AIDS control is made part of PHC, the cost is simply too prohibitive for many countries to bear by themselves. The worldwide control of the AIDS epidemic requires international cooperation.

The first step, of course, is careful planning of programs at the community level. Every effort should be made to use existing structures and facilities to cut costs. Volunteers should be recruited and trained to provide needed services. Carefully designed budgets should be developed and efforts made to raise money locally. Concurrently, attempts should be made to solicit money outside the community and country.

In many African countries, churches and political parties have raised funds through "harvest festivals." This is a sort of auction whereby local people send products from the farm or store-bought items to be sold. The church or party organizes the festival, where people bid on various items usually at a price much higher than market value. The church or party uses the money raised for needed activities. Harvest festivals and other traditional ways of raising money should be used in some of these countries to raise needed funds for AIDS control. In U.S. black communities, the church could be a major force in fund-raising activities. Other political and civic groups could also help. School and university students may embark on various fund-raising activities.

Raising money outside the community should involve active and passive solicitation. Local AIDS activity agencies should seek out and solicit funds from governmental and nongovernmental organizations at regional and national levels. Such nongovernmental organizations as foundations, corporations, and churches should be aggressively pursued. On the other hand, these organizations could simply donate money and equipment to community-based AIDS activity agencies.

International governmental and nongovernmental agencies are particularly needed for AIDS activity funding in African and other Third World countries. Countries such as the United States and Japan, western European countries, and oil-rich gulf countries are in a position to make substantial contributions. Perhaps it would be too expensive for one or a few of these countries to donate needed funds, but, if all or most of them contributed, the burden would be less unbearable. The process of solicitation should be the same as described in the last paragraph. These countries may also donate equipment and supplies, drugs, and experts in addition to money. How the money and supplies are used should be determined at the local level with input from international agencies.

The scope of the AIDS epidemic is already enormous and is likely to widen. Aggressive and quick control activities are needed to prevent a very bad situation from getting worse. The task appears insurmountable; the costs appear to be prohibitive; and there are no simple answers. But the world cannot afford to ignore the problem. We cannot afford to let whole populations die. With political commitment, long and careful planning, and total community involvement, the AIDS epidemic can be controlled despite the world economic situation. In a speech on the implementation of primary health care, the former Director General of WHO, Dr. Halden Mahler, said: "The goal is there; the ways to attain it are daily becoming clearer; and . . . if we temper our dreams with realism we shall reach our goal in spite of the world's political and economic malaise" (Bolard & Young, 1982, p. 241).

## REFERENCE

Bolard, R. G. A., & Young, M. E. M. (1982). The strategy, costs, and progress of primary health care. *Bulletin of the Pan American Health Organization, 16*, 233-241.

# About the Author

Samuel V. Duh (M.D., M.P.H.) is Medical Executive Director of the Flagler County Health Department in Florida. His medical degree is from the University of North Carolina, Chapel Hill, and he did his postdoctoral training, in internal medicine, preventive medicine, and public health, at the University of Oklahoma, the Montefiore Hospital in Pittsburgh, and the Texas Department of Health in Austin. Prior to his current position, he worked in several public health settings and in clinical practice in Texas. He has made numerous presentations at local, national, and international meetings on AIDS. His articles have appeared in the *Journal of the American Medical Association, Journal of the National Medical Association, Archives of Internal Medicine,* and *Public Health Reports.*